DR. RODICA MALOS

The TRUTH UN-MASKED

Never Again

The TRUTH UN-MASKED

Never Again

How Authorities Silenced Doctors
Who Embraced Truth and Freedom
and Saved Lives During the Pandemic

DR. RODICA MALOS
DNP, ANP, GNP, BSN, RN, Ec.

The Truth Un-masked – Never Again

ISBN NR. 979-8-89814-278-0

Published by: Lascau Scriptum Ministries INC.
8489 W. Heather CT, Glendale, AZ 85305
Phone (602) 291-0175 – www.Lascauscriptum.com

Cover: Rodica Lascau

*"Yes, and all who desire
to live godly in Christ Jesus
will suffer persecution."*

2 Timothy 3:12

*"And you shall know the truth,
and the truth shall make you free."*

John 8:32

*The highest honor and the highest call
of every human being on this planet
is to stand up for the truth
and to fight for freedom.
Persecution for the truth is real.*

Dr. Rodica Malos

Disclaimer

This book contains the opinions and ideas of the author. It is solely for informational and educational purposes and should not be regarded as a substitute for professional medical treatment. The nature of your body's health condition is complex and unique. Therefore, you should consult a health professional before you begin any new lifestyle change, exercise, nutrition, fasting, or supplementation program, or if you have questions about your health.

Neither the author nor the publisher shall be liable or responsible for any loss or damage allegedly arising from any information or suggestions in this book. People and names in this book are composites created by the author from her experiences as a primary care practitioner. Names and details of their stories have been changed, and any similarity between the names and stories of individuals described in this book and individuals known to readers is purely coincidental. The statements in this book about consumable products or food have not been evaluated by the Food and Drug Administration. The recipes in this book are to be followed exactly as written.

The publisher is not responsible for your specific health or allergy needs that may require medical supervision. The publisher is not responsible for any adverse reactions to the consumption of food or products that have been suggested in this book. While the author has made every effort to provide accurate internet addresses at the time of publication, neither the publisher nor the author assumes any responsibility for errors or for changes that occur after publication. Further, the publisher does not have any control over and does not assume any responsibility for author or third-party websites or their content.

Endorsements for THE TRUTH UN-MASKED

I had the privilege and honor of meeting Dr. Rodica Malos at the Romanian Parliament in Bucharest, Romania—her native country—during the International Covid Summit (ICS) in 2023. We then met again the following year in Washington, DC at CPAC/ICS. Dr. Malos is an extraordinary woman, a brave doctor, and an exemplary human being. In a time when truth was stifled, courage became the rarest and most valuable commodity. Dr. Malos delivers a powerful, firsthand account of the battle for medical freedom, human rights, and the ethical duty of physicians to put their patients first—no matter what the cost. Through personal sacrifice and unwavering conviction, this book serves as both a warning and a call to action for all who cherish liberty.

With a deep understanding of both authoritarian control and the sanctity of freedom, Dr. Malos shares a gripping narrative that is as much a personal journey as it is a historical record of an era that must never be forgotten. This book is not just a reflection on the past—it is a guide for the future, urging us to stand firm in our principles, even in the face of overwhelming adversity. A must-read for anyone who values truth, freedom, and the courage to stand against the tide.

--Dr. Alejandro Diaz
Pediatric Allergist-Immunologist &
Global Health Specialist

In this remarkably prescient book, Dr. Rodica Malos sets a timeless appeal to stand up in a culture of lies and distortion of the truth. I cannot imagine a more timely and urgent book full of insightful and spiritual truth. This book is a counsel of hope for even the bleakest days and encouragement we need, especially in today's cascading times.

--Shaneen Clarke, London, England
Author, The Lord of the Silence

During the COVID-19 years, few medical providers did the right thing. Many refused to look at the straightforward medical facts. Namely, that there were early treatments that worked and that lockdowns were harmful. Most just complied with their employers—a more subtle version of "just following orders." In 2020, I founded America's Frontline Doctors to stand against the propaganda of the "public health establishment." Since then, I have sought out those freedom warriors who are unafraid to speak the truth. Dr. Rodica Malos is such a person. As an immigrant from a communist nation, she recognized the authoritarian infrastructure that has unfortunately taken hold in America. Her story is important, insightful, and inspiring.

--Dr. Simone Gold, MD, JD
Founder, AFLDS.org and CEO, GoldCare.com

Dr. Malos has stood shoulder to shoulder with us as we stood up for medical freedom, and against the evil that threatened to destroy our humanity as we know it. So many have forgotten the price we paid. So many have forgotten what happened in 2020 as global governments turned against the very people they were supposed to protect. So many doctors and patriots lost jobs, licenses, and businesses as we collectively refused to comply to autocracy disguised as medicine. The book digs into the price many paid and serves as a reminder to humanity. Never forget! Dr. Malos is a colleague and thankfully a sister in Christ. This is a must-read.

--Dr. Stella Immanuel, MD
Physician, author, international speaker,
entrepreneur and minister of the gospel

Dr. Rodica Malos reminds us of the ultimate truth given to us by God: "Howbeit when he, the Spirit of truth, is come, he will guide you into all truth: for he shall not speak of himself; but whatsoever he shall hear, that shall he speak: and he will shew you things to come"(John 16:13 KJV).

Dr. Malos wrote The Cost For Truth to remind us about the past persecution she faced under the dictatorship of the authoritarian Romanian government during the communist regime in the country of her origin. And, now here in the United States. She is speaking truth directly from the Holy Spirit as a guiding light by placing a spotlight on governmental overreach of power, which restricted freedom in providing care to suffering people. This created fear and psychological distress, affecting the lives of many. This book is a wake-up call to learn why truth from the ultimate source is vital to circumvent another horrible event in global healthcare.

People of all generations need to learn about the tyrannical methods used by the enemy to silence courageous clinicians who chose to stand up for the truth and who embraced freedom in medicine to provide patient-centered care to save lives at any cost. We owe it to the Lord Jesus Christ for providing the ultimate tools of how to stand against spiritual and physical persecution, as explained in this book. As Paul wrote to the Corinthians: "For the weapons of our warfare are not carnal, but mighty through God to the pulling down of strong holds" (2 Cor. 10:4 KJV).

This work is a must read! Well done!

--Dr. Avery M. Jackson III MD, Neurosurgeon
Trustee, The Body Healthcare
Founder, Great Lakes Learning
Author, The God Prescription

Dr. Rodica Malos is a voice for the nations to help both warn and encourage with faith. Through her personal story, we discover there is real hope for us through Jesus Christ and His servants who will not remain silent, but instead stand up and fight for liberty and freedom. I met Dr. Malos in Washington State in USA when I was speaking at a conference. The first time I met her I could sense her tenacity and desire to see people saved, healed, delivered, and set free. She has remained consistent in this fervor for the health of humanity with the release of The CostFor Truth. Let us learn what is necessary to propel forward so we as a culture do not make the same mistakes again. Thank you, Dr. Malos!

--Dr. Candice Smithyman
Founder, Dream Mentors International
Author, speaker, host of Glory Road TV Show

"I just finished reading this book this morning and I have to say it's the best! I loved Dr. Malos's understanding and use of the scriptures to continue the undergirding of everything she writes. It is what gives the book life and supernatural power beyond information and wisdom. This kind of commitment to the truth, both clinically and spiritually, is life-giving and so needed in this current generation and culture.

I was especially blessed with the inclusion of the church as integral in the healing and sustaining health for people. I know there are a lot of "self-help" books on the market but real hope—the hope that Dr. Malos writes about—is truly the product of the life found in God and the salvation freely offered to all through Jesus Christ! I am praying that God will use this book to set captives free and open hearts, but most of all to reintroduce Jesus to all who with open hearts read her story and are looking for hope in a broken world.

I highly recommend this book. It is filled with gems of life, even though I shed a tear or two as I read the tragic stories of those who lost loved ones, fought through their recovery, and continue to face lingering effects of COVID-19. Thank you, Dr. Rodica, for not keeping silent! You are a true warrior for truth in the seen and unseen eternal realms!

On a personal note, I want to thank Dr. Malos once again for saving my life after my diagnosis of COVID-19. With a history of heart issues, I am certain the protocols she encouraged me to follow helped me recover and continue to enjoy my life, family and the ministry God has given Lisa and me!

--Senior Pastor Brad (and Lisa) Makowski
Anthem Church, Fairview, Oregon

In her new book, Dr. Rodica Malos shares with all of us some very unfortunate experiences she encountered during the COVID-19 pandemic, in order to prevent them from happening again in the future. That time period was difficult and troubling for all of us. But as we learn from Dr. Malos, the situation got much worse for members of Frontline Doctors, who simply wanted to provide the best care and treatment for their patients.

Writing from her unique perspective as a born-again believer, a doctor, and an immigrant from a communist country where she witnessed persecution firsthand, the author exposes many hard-to-believe realities taking place in a developed nation, boasting top performance in critical areas of health care.

The word persecution is used in this book repeatedly, not only in reference to the actions of the authoritarian Romanian government of the 1970s and '80s, but surprisingly in reference to the actions of the government, here in the "land of the free." Throughout Dr. Malos's book, you will read about the governmental interference and restricted freedom of speech, thought, and expression here in the United States. Pretending they were for the health and safety of the public, many rights were cancelled during the early days of the pandemic. It is our responsibility as citizens to learn from what took place during the COVID-19 pandemic and help educate future generations.

My wife and I are also Romanians who escaped communist oppression in the early 1980s and emigrated to the United States to enjoy religious freedom. We believe it is very important for all of us to sound the alarm when the basic rights of people are being limited in any part of the world.

Congratulations to our dear friend, Dr. Rodica Malos, for writing this book. We are convinced that it will benefit many people in generations to come.

--Rev. Vasile (and Rodica) Cinpean
Lead Pastor, Philadelphia Romanian Church, Portland, Oregon
President, Romanian Alliance Fellowship, Assemblies of God USA

We are very thankful for the deep resolve that Dr. Rodica and her husband made to stand for truth and freedom in the medical field. That decision saved the lives of so many and will continue for many generations to come. We are most grateful, for we are two of the lives that Dr. Rodica's medical care saved! We pray that justice for persecuted doctors for saving lives will be restored and that they will be able to continue with the highest calling of their lives.

--Pastors Ed & Cheryl Rebman
DWF New Beginnings Stream Church, Portland, Oregon

Dr. Rodica Malos has opened the depths of the surgical wound of our Covid pandemic and through her personal experiences has laid bare the pathway forward to examine the truth behind our current public health crisis. She has challenged us to look carefully at all scientific breakthroughs, protocols, and mandates with new eyes. We must never stop asking and seeking the best practices that render the most efficient and compassionate care available worldwide.

We have much to learn from her perspective on government mandates, persecution, and overreach from her days living in communist Romania to her practitioner days in the United States. Let us always stand for doing the right thing, even if it means sacrifice and persecution. May her testimony reach the ears of all in the medical profession and the legislative bodies governing health policies.

May we never forget the wrongs done to our fellow human beings and strive to always fight for the right outcomes for our family, clients, patients, children, and future generations. God bless Dr. Rodica Malos for her ongoing war and may the Frontline Doctors'—who are waiting for the restoration of justice—licenses be reestablished.

--Kay E. Metsger R.N. BSN
Former cardiac operating room nurse manager
Providence St. Vincent Medical Center, Portland, Oregon

We hear that the strongest people of character are those who are refined like gold in the fire of adversity. I am so honored to have been a witness to a living example of the golden character I have seen in Dr. Rodica Malos. In the high-stress times of treating patients during the pandemic, like many doctors on the front lines, she was caught in the crossfire of having to choose between her license and the lives of her patients. She chose to save lives. Countless testimonials of patients and their families attest to her research and dedication keeping her patients out of the hospital and from near-death experiences in the height of highly restrictive practices.

The many stories of Frontline Doctors choosing to save lives, which they did very successfully—while colliding with restrictive protocols—cost them their careers despite doing good and no harm. Many people can relate to times when doing the right thing is doing a hard thing. I have seen many doctors choose to love people, live above offense, and continue to study and thrive in the area of their expertise. Doctors who kept their oath to serve their patients rather than to themselves, and follow their conscience, not the crowd.

I speak for the literally hundreds of thousands of lives they touched with true compassion during a time that was highly stressful for all of us. Thank you, Rodica, for sharing your great mind for research and your heart of refined gold.

--Laura Rau, Retired RN Case Manager
Executive director of Stress Management and Recovery Program
Legacy Mt. Hood Medical Center, Gresham, Oregon

Dr. Rodica has bravely pioneered a path that each of us, in various ways and intensities, will walk if we are to fully give our lives over to our Lord and Savior, Jesus Christ. This path is one of zero compromise and extreme courage in the face of the spirit of fear. It is the path of choosing God, choosing courage, choosing love and truth at the cost of worldly possessions, titles and human accolades. This book will infuse you with courage!

--Jenny Donnelly
Founder, Her Voice Movement
#DontMessWithOurKids-USA

The author, Dr. Rodica Malos, made immense sacrifices in her unwavering fight for the truth. She gave her time, health, and even her so-hard-to-achieve medical license in pursuit of justice and integrity. Her story inspires us all to stand firm in our convictions, regardless the cost. As Paul wrote to the Colossians: "Now I rejoice in what I am suffering for you, and I fill up in my flesh what is still lacking in regard to Christ's afflictions, for the sake of his body, which is the church" (Col. 1:24 NIV).

Paul was not implying that Christ's sufferings on the cross were insufficient for salvation. Rather, he sees his own sufferings as a continuation of Christ's work in the world for building up and supporting the church. That is exactly what this book is all about. The Cost of Standing For All Generations masterfully intertwines three scenarios, each intricately linked in a balanced way: 1) the COVID plague: a harrowing depiction of death and despair amidst the absence of adequate prevention and medical treatment; 2) the atrocities of communism with firsthand accounts of suffering and oppression endured under a communist regime, 3) the fight against evil—a relentless struggle against darkness, culminating in the ultimate sovereignty of God, the Creator of the universe.

As John 14:6 says, Jesus Christ, the Son of God, is "the way, the truth, and the life."

The outcome of the fight against evil is life—life for countless thousands of people. For some, the victory brings a profound opportunity to share the goodness of God, spreading hope and faith. For others, it serves as a chance to repent and humbly submit to the Creator of life, embracing His sovereignty and grace. The narrative emphasizes the eminence of impending events, urging readers to be prepared. A thought-provoking question resonates throughout the story: Which path do you choose to belong to?

--Dr. Mihaela Beloiu, MD, Senior Doctor
Family practice specialty
Millennium Physician Group
Palmetto, Florida

ACKNOWLEDGMENTS

This book received support from the Creator of the universe, who gave the world supernatural prescriptions in His living Word to overcome fear and to manage high levels of stress, anxiety, and depression during pandemic time and every day in life. I thank Jesus Christ, the Lamb of God, and the Lord and Savior of my life and the entire world. He delivers those who believe in Him from the stress of sin and from all their fears in any situation, including pandemic time. Only He restores the joy of salvation and gives hope and peace. The peace that passes all understanding and guards their minds, spirits, and bodies during this pandemic period.

I acknowledge the Holy Spirit, the great Comforter, who literally guided me through every step in treating patients with symptoms from COVID-19 and in writing this book. He is the power of God working on earth, giving to those who ask Him inspiration, wisdom, knowledge, revelation, and discernment to cope with high levels of stress, fear, anxiety, and depression. Also, I give millions of thanks to my beloved husband, Stelica, for his sacrifices, support, encouragement, and love during the pandemic. Especially while I was involved in so many extra hours, helping the most vulnerable people suffering from symptoms of COVID-19 at every level. Millions of thanks to my entire family, including the in-laws who worked in health care on the front lines, providing care relentlessly and tirelessly to patients suffering from many kinds of diseases during the pandemic; they made great sacrifices. I give many thanks to friends, colleagues, and all my patients who were in my sphere of influence, and who provided support and inspiration throughout the entire pandemic.

Many thanks to all the writers, doctors, experts and scientists cited in this book and all those standing for the truth and the churches (I call them "spiritual clinics") that continued to pray fervently for those in great need of healing. You sacrificed your time to make the information available to inspire me and the entire community. We benefit from the scientific evidence and your spiritual insights. You change our thinking and motivate us to have a better lifestyle, to live a quality life here on earth and for eternity. Special thanks to Mr. Ken Walker, the editor, for helping me finish and publish this book.

Special thanks to you for reading the information in this book, with the hope that it will enrich your knowledge and will give a new perspective for life on this planet and in eternity. It will strengthen your spirit, renew your mind and thoughts, improve your physical and spiritual health, and prevent physical and spiritual diseases.

Many thanks as well to Dr. Robert Sayson and all Frontline Doctors who sacrificed their profession, including Drs. Jill and Robert Malone. They played a huge role in this project by inviting me to the ICS-4 to participate and speak at the Romanian Parliament in Bucharest in 2023, and then to ICS-5 and CPAC in Washington, DC in 2024, which led me to write this book. You both are giants of faith—fighting for freedom, standing up for the truth, and tirelessly traveling the entire world to impact all generations with the truth.

Dedication

To my three sweet grandchildren—Jude, Liam, and Stella—who through their appearance in this world brought deep insights about God's creation, beholding the most powerful miracles in the entire universe and the most precious gifts from heaven. Since their birth, I have been holding and am looking at God's marvelous work. A work of invisible things bringing into existence the human body. With them, every single cell functions, based on God's programming through His breath and His Holy Spirit's energy since creation. God created the first DNA that carries hereditary material packed in the genes, which gives every single person unique features in "the seed" placed by God from creation, with the power to multiply exponentially. To my faithful and lovely husband, Stely (married for almost four decades), and our only daughter, Dr. Andreea Steward, PharmD, and our son-in-law, Jeff, who truly love God and magnify the Lord Jesus and His Holy Spirit in their lives. I thank God for each one of you. With the Lord on our side, we overcame numerous obstacles to be where we are today. I appreciate your huge sacrifices. I love each one of you tremendously.

Table of Contents

Foreword

I witnessed firsthand the Frontline Doctors, including Dr. Rodica Malos, who persevered through stressful trials and persecution. They faced opposition simply for standing up for the truth and fighting for freedom in medicine at any cost. Because the love of God compelled her to care and stand for truth during the COVID-19 pandemic, Dr. Malos had to pay a high price—like many other doctors who faced persecution for the "crime" of saving lives. She dared to provide compassionate, evidence-based first line care for suffering patients. Patients who were bewildered by being sent home from the ER or not being able to be seen by any provider. The health system's mantra was "stay home, sicken in place, and go to the ER only when you get worse."

Health authorities made no mention of any kind of helpful remedy. But Dr. Malos diligently searched available literature for incoming information. She also contacted leading doctors who were gaining valuable experience treating patients on the front lines, and reporting successful measures that they had observed. She risked her own health to see and follow up with her patients. That included even doing occasional home visits to reassure them and ensure that they were getting the best available care. Based on the experience of many other providers finding positive results, her advice and off-label use of medications to treat her COVID-19 patients resulted in most of them getting rapidly better at home. That is expressed in their notes of gratitude, which you will read in this book.

The persecutions for standing up for the truth in medicine and for providing care to suffering patients from symptoms from a lethal pathogen reminded her of what she had experienced in Communist Romania and its "intimidation" practices to enforce fear, dictatorship, and tyranny. That is one reason she was so troubled about the same thing happening in the USA, the "land of the free."

The governmental overreach of power restricted freedom of clinical judgment and thinking process in providing care to suffering people, many sentenced to die from a lethal pathogen. Using the pretext of "public safety," the rights of people around the world were cancelled, leaving them to live in fear and psychological distress. The society had to suffer from lies and propaganda that affected the economy, education, and physical and mental health, with a negative impact for generations. This book is a wake-up call to this generation and all generations to come—to learn about unbelievable inhumane approaches in medicine and do not let them happen again in the future.

People of all generations need to learn about the tyrannical methods used to silence members of Frontline Doctors who chose to stand up for the truth and embraced freedom in medicine. All to provide patient-centered care and save their lives at any cost. May all of us educate this generation and future generations to not allow the same tyranny to happen again. The voice of the author clearly resounds in this book: NEVER AGAIN.

These losses and mandates experienced by the Front Line doctors through their persecutions severely handicapped community health centers from caring for the poor and uninsured in all communities. I believe this insightful book by Dr. Malos will bless many by opening their eyes to the harm that was done during the pandemic. Especially by lockdowns initiated in an effort to control people through fear and suppression of truth. Dr. Malos shows us how to discern the times and respond with truth and love. She prepares us all for a future time of persecution by modeling how to persevere with hope, truth and love. Jesus declared in Mark 13:13, "You will be hated by all for My name's sake. But he who endures to the end shall be saved." Hebrews 12:11 states, "For the moment, all discipline seems painful rather than pleasant, but later it yields the peaceful fruit of righteousness to those who have been trained by it" (ESV).

Let us all draw encouragement from those words.

--Dr. Robert Sayson, MD
Acting Medical Director
Good News Community Health Center
Portland, Oregon

INTRODUCTION

Persecution for the truth was real during the communist regime in the country of my origin and is real today in the "land of the free." Fighting for freedom is everyone's duty, to prevent communism from resurfacing, along with dictatorship, totalitarianism, globalism, and the consequences of losing our freedom for generations to come. Reflecting on what happened under communist dictatorship and the tyranny that took place in medicine in the last five years, the question, "What did I do?", led me to write this book. I wanted to bring more awareness to those who read that we must stand up for the truth and for freedom for the next generations. We must not let the same catastrophes happen again in the future, no matter how hard it will be to do the right thing.

The same question should motivate us all to keep fighting for the truth to the end, even though we may face persecution at the hands of the dictators in charge of the various establishments that govern our lives: "What did you do?"

"Patients first" was the mandate persisting in healthcare professionals' mind in the entire health care system. And, in my mind as a healthcare provider in different roles for more than three decades in the US. But during pandemic time, everything changed. During the pandemic, the inhuman behavior of dictators banning treatment for patients suffering from Covid and the persecution of doctors who saved lives shook humanity to the core. It also led me to write this book as a reminder to not let this kind of disaster to ever happen again. I repeat here what I say in chapter 22: NEVER AGAIN.

When patients suffering from symptoms from Covid needed the most attention from primary care providers, they were lied to and told there was "no treatment." Then they were sent home with no treatment, abandoned, and sentenced to live with the fear of dying alone in isolation, with nobody at their side to hold their hands. That lie was a big disservice to US citizens and the entire world's population. Such tyranny should never happen again.

Professionals who had been trained in the most prominent medical schools, hospitals, clinics, and specialty departments to take care of patients when they were suffering from different acute and chronic symptoms and diagnoses found themselves helpless to offer solutions. This during a time when suffering patients needed them the most.

Symptoms from COVID-19 were treatable conditions with safe, effective, and affordable medication. But the lack of guidelines for primary care practitioners to treat early acute symptoms from this deadly virus posed a nightmare for doctors on the front lines. It was a very sinister situation, knowing that the treatable inflammatory process from coronavirus damaged patients' lungs. Some patients ended up on ventilators and others died prematurely (and unnecessarily).

Meditating on the tyranny of letting patients suffer with no early treatment made me extremely uncomfortable. The idea of staying relaxed as a primary care provider and "doing nothing"—per authorities' recommendation to let patients suffer until their symptoms got worse and only then go to the hospital? I couldn't abide by that, so I made the decision to keep my promise of offering "patient-centered care." I would stand up for the truth to provide appropriate care for such a time as this. But like many others in Frontline Doctors, I had to pay a very high price, which I describe in this book.

Frontline Doctors who embraced truth and freedom in medicine were threatened by medical establishments with the loss of their licenses and their careers. They were censored and their character assassinated as they faced humiliation and persecution for the "crime" of saving lives. Even President Trump was humiliated by mainstream media when he stood up for the truth. Numerous outlets ridiculed him for suggesting early treatment was accessible with hydroxychloroquine, even prophylactically, to save people's lives. The media silenced the president of the United States with their lies, negative reports, and criticism. In essence, they left the entire country with no hope, tormented by fear caused by manipulative propaganda.

Millions could have learned from the president's experience with prophylactic treatment and the Frontline Doctors, with so much expertise in primary care management in treating these people, and so many others like them. Early treatment could have prevented hospitalization and further damage done by this virus. It harmed people physically, emotionally, socially, and economically, affecting people's quality of life and leading many to a premature death.

The president of the USA did not keep silent, though. He cried out to tell the truth to the American people and the world that there was hope. He disclosed to the public that he was taking HCQ and encouraged the American people (who were rightly scared by this unpredictable and aggressive virus) to take it prophylactically, as he did as a preventative measure. He was right in presenting HCQ as being an antidote for COVID-19 for the majority of the USA population—if taken early, before their symptoms worsened. We had a leader who did not keep silent and was disclosing the truth from his personal experience so that many other lives could be saved. But just like the Frontline Doctors, the media silenced the president by accusing him of "spreading misinformation."

As this battle unfolded, I often felt like David facing Goliath. Still, I knew that David won the battle with the giant because he had God on his side. With that picture in mind, I began the battle by finding a "Hiding Place" for my suffering patients at Good News Clinic so their lives could be saved from the "holocaust" caused by the virus. That's what Dutch author Corrie ten Boom called the small room her father created in their house to hide Jewish people from being arrested by the Gestapo secret police during World War II's Holocaust. Standing up for the truth and freedom for the next generations is the highest call for us all, even if we need to pay a very high price. We must fight for freedom for our children's children.

Chapter 1

Grace Under Fire

The story you're about to read concerns maintaining grace in the crucible of injustice, irrational decisions, and stunning persecution. Most of all, it is a story about faith. The faith that sustained me though the lockdowns of the pandemic and many agonizing months that followed. The repercussions of this frightening experience have lasted to this day. Yet faith in my Lord and Savior, Jesus Christ, has helped me endure the same kind of persecution I faced growing up in Romania under stifling, overbearing, godless communist rule. That I experienced similar opposition in a free land is a bit saddening, yet not surprising. No matter where we live, we will always face leaders who want to lord it over us, govern our daily choices and decisions, and prove that they have ultimate power.

That I withstood some of the worst pressure imaginable is a praise to the Lord. Generally, nobody welcomes persecution and tribulations. But fellowship with Christ's suffering takes place when we are going through trials, investigations, and persecutions. This is the time we draw closest to Him in our prayer and petitions. It is when we have a special communion with Him who suffered for us first. We must go through various trials to be closer to Christ.

It is a Christian formula to pray and participate in the rite of Communion with other believers, when we are asked to remember Christ's suffering together. In persecutions and trials our reputation is often adversely affected; we can suffer overwhelming distress and discouragement. But Jesus said to rejoice in those moments. As James wrote: "Count it joy when you fall into various trials, knowing that the testing of your faith produces patience" (James 1:2–3).

This passage from James changed my perspective during a painful time, when I grieved over losing my nurse practitioner's license after so many years of completing education and enjoying the rich experiences offered by primary care medicine. After living through this devastating time, I assure everyone reading this: we cannot allow this to happen again.

Frightening Flashback

It's been more than five years since the draconian lockdowns rippled across the world and created fear, suspicion, and division that has lived with us since that awful day. A day that began in January of 2020 in China and spread to the United States by mid-March. But there was something equally insidious going on in the months that followed. Doctors were persecuted for daring to deviate from the government line, telling the truth, or prescribing certain medications that could save lives. I know, because it eventually cost me my license as a primary care provider.

That this could happen in the "land of the free and the home of the brave" is especially frightening. Growing up in Romania, I had seen up close the horrors of an authoritarian government that exerts pressure over its citizens' lives, determining what they can do, where they can live, how many children they can bear, and how they can make a living. This was my nightmarish existence in my native land of Romania.

My past is one reason I believe so strongly in freedom, the right of people to be free from governmental interference in their lives, and the right to freedom of speech, freedom of thought, and freedom of expression. Under the guise of health and safety during the early days of the pandemic, all those rights were suppressed and in some ways still are. I sound the alarm to inform and alert our citizens to the threats they face now and in days to come.

A Lethal Pathogen

When the horrors of the pandemic unfolded, interventions that saved lives during the onset of Covid-19 wound up getting banned. That left primary care providers with no weapons to fight a lethal pathogen that killed millions of people worldwide. The lack of guidelines for primary care practitioners to treat early acute symptoms from this deadly virus posed a nightmare for doctors on the front lines of treatment. People who had been trained in prominent medical schools, hospitals, clinics, and specialty departments to take care of patients when they were suffering from different acute and chronic symptoms and diagnoses found themselves helpless to offer solutions. During lockdowns, when patients needed the most attention from primary care providers, they were sent home with no treatment. They felt abandoned and sentenced to live with the fear of dying alone in isolation, with nobody at their side to hold their hands. Today as I reflect on that nightmare, I sometimes ask myself if the freedom to live has been lost.

Emotions of sadness gripped my heart and thoughts of desperations ran through my mind as I thought of the past. Especially memories of my parents telling my brothers and sisters and I about their struggles, suffering, and persecution as they ran from secret police to preserve their lives during World War II in Europe, both during the Holocaust and the communist takeover that followed. They lived a life of sacrifices so we, their children and the generations to follow, would be safe and face an optimistic future.

The spirit of compassion for those hopeless patients when Covid began overwhelmed my heart. I have always had compassion for suffering patients from any condition, so the deadly virus that suddenly engulfed the world gave me new determination to do the right thing. I had to stay upright, tell the truth, and put my patients first. I had to expend my energies and give unselfishly to save their lives.

As this battle unfolded, I felt like David facing Goliath. Still, I knew that David won the battle with the giant because he had God on his side. With that picture in mind I began the battle by finding a "Hiding Place." That's what Dutch author Corrie ten Boom called the small room her father created in their house to hide Jewish people from being arrested by the Gestapo secret police during the Holocaust. Standing up for the truth and freedom for the next generation is the highest call for us all, even if we need to pay a very high price. We must fight for freedom for our children's children.

Standing for Truth

Returning from the Conservative Political Action Conference (CPAC) in February of 2024, my heart surged with emotion. All the speakers who had stood up for truth and freedom for the next generations had moved my heart. So did their messages begging the audience of thousands of people to do the same for the sake of their children, grandchildren, and great-grandchildren. They stirred a resolve deep in my heart to not give up fighting for freedom in medicine, all for the sake of generations to come.

I also felt overwhelmed as I reflected on what happened over the past year, with my license revocation in April of 2023 by heavy-handed health care authorities in my state. These people had been unmoved by the fact that I had saved countless lives during the pandemic by volunteering my time at a small clinic in our area, serving minorities and the most vulnerable among us.

That would be followed by an invitation from Frontline Doctors to attend their White Coat Summit in Washington, DC at the Supreme Court (July of 2023), where I met like-minded experts, doctors, clinicians, scientists, and political leaders. In Washington I received an invitation from Dr. Robert Malone to attend the International Crisis Summit IV at the Romanian Parliament in Bucharest. Held in November of 2023, the forum featured top medical experts, analysts, scientists, health care providers, and political leaders. While there I received an invitation to CPAC's meeting in February of 2024.

Everything happened so fast that I struggled to find the time to review the data and information from all the great speakers I had heard. I like to know what is going on in the world and how the victims of propaganda and censorship are affected by current events. I also enjoy meeting the heroes and persecuted doctors and medical experts for standing up for truth and fighting for freedom in the health care field.

The "Free Book"

During a short break between sessions at CPAC, I was threading my way through the crowd and up the stairs to the coffee shop. Suddenly I noticed a nice young woman looking at me intensely. She raised one hand with a book in it, insisting I could have it "for free." I hesitated, but she kept insisting. One reason for my hesitancy came from the fact that just looking at another title made my head spin. I had already read so many books about the pandemic and the attendant injustices, totalitarianism, and lies spread by authorities. This material made me reflect again about persecution for telling the truth in a free world and stirred deep emotions within.

So did reliving those moments when I took matters into my own hands and started to treat early pandemic sufferers. These were desperate people in agony, knowing they were close to the grave. I talked to them every single day until I knew they had recovered or were at least out of danger. I could literally feel their agony deep in my soul. The unpleasant moments when I faced intimidation from the health care establishment also stung my heart. Imagine being investigated for the "crime" of treating suffering patients.

All of this swirled through my mind while this beautiful woman insisted I take the book from her outstretched hand. I thought that if I read another book with some painful information I should at least pay something. But when I tried to take some money from wallet, she insisted on giving it to me. After pushing it into my hand, she vanished into the crowd. I never saw her again.

Ironically, I wanted to pay even though I felt ill-prepared to read another book about the war against humans during Covid, post-Covid, and long-Covid lockdowns, facemasks, and vaccine mandates. In addition to acting as a primary care provider, I became a victim of the virus. For sharing the protocols with those desperate for solutions, the state stripped me of my license as a general practitioner.

Because that anonymous woman insisted that I take it, I now held in my hands another book chronicling catastrophes against humanity. It sickened me, even though I had already read many books written by doctors standing up for the truth and sacrificing their profession, career, and licenses because of tyranny during the pandemic. Established medical authorities allowed patients to die without early treatment, at a time when they needed it the most.

A Broken Heart

I reflected often in those early days of the pandemic and how people who relied on doctors, nurses, and professional health care providers were abandoned. We let them die when we could have taken simple steps to use safe, off-label medications that we had used for decades for various symptoms. Like anti-inflammatory medications for inflammation in patients' lungs, anti-viral medications for viral infections, antibiotics for secondary bronchitis and pneumonia, bronchodilators and steroids via nebulizers for respiratory problems, or anti-thrombolytic for blood clots. Even prophylactic treatments are usually used in certain situations in medicine. I thought, "Why is it impossible now to use the same approach to save people's lives and protect them from this enemy? Why should we let them live in fear of dying unnecessarily?"

Such questions absolutely broke my heart. Even as I write this book, tears run down my face as I think about the numerous young patients who died prematurely (and unnecessarily), leaving behind wives, husbands, children, parents, and relatives. I have close relatives and friends who are still grieving for their loved ones. It is likely their emotional pain will never heal.

I also feel sick over the treatment my husband and I suffered when the coronavirus struck us and our primary care providers told my husband and me: "There is no treatment for Covid." Simply put, they lied to us. I knew that all my patients whom I treated with early interventions recovered and are alive today because I was willing to step out of my comfort zone. When patients suffer, you must do everything possible to alleviate their pain, make them feel better, and save their lives.

Facing Two Wars

Our patients, including my husband and myself, were fighting two wars. A physical war when our body was infected with a lethal pathogen even after receiving the mandated vaccinations. It hit us physically to the core, causing weakness, lethargy, lack of energy, and respiratory problems. We also battled emotional distress when our doctors told us there was no treatment for symptoms from Covid. We felt as if we had been sentenced to die.

As soon as CPAC concluded, my husband and I had to leave. Fortunately, on my computer I had Kindle access to read books that I had begun earlier during the six-hour flight from Washington, DC to Portland. I had decided to not touch any "heavy" books during this time. I did not want to have to reflect on yet another book filled with information that would remind me of the painful catastrophes of recent months. But as soon as we got seated on our flight, I found myself reaching for the "free book."

As I read, I came to a pivotal paragraph. It jumped out at me and grabbed me with the force of someone gripping my throat: "Someday all our kids and grandkids will ask each of us directly: 'Why did you stand by? Why did you not help me? I could not breathe.' Or God forbid: 'Now I have these health problems.' Or else they will say:

'Thank you so much for speaking for me when I was too little to speak.' 'Dad, Mom, Grandma, Grandpa,' they will ask: 'What did you do?' So let me leave you with this question: What did you do?"[1]

That question stirred my heart: "What did I do?" It prompted me to start thinking more about what I should do. A verse from Proverbs immediately came to mind: "A good man leaves an inheritance to his children's children" (Prov. 13:22). In my mind pictures emerged: sick parents who were desperate for treatment, grateful that I was able to save them from premature death. But then other sad images came to mind, like a young family with six children; both parents died from Covid a few months apart, leaving behind those beautiful children. Or another family of thirteen children, all grieving the loss of their father to Covid at thirty-nine years of age, with only their mother to provide for them.

That question, "What did I do?" led me to write this book to bring more awareness to those who read that we must stand up for the truth and for the freedom for the next generations. We must not let the same catastrophes to happen again in the future, no matter how hard it will be to do the right thing.

The same question should motivate us to keep fighting for the truth to the end, even though we may face persecution at the hands of the dictators in charge of the various establishments that govern our lives: "What did you do?" As John wrote in his prophetic book: "Here is the patience of the saints; here are those who keep the commandments of God and the faith of Jesus" (Rev. 14:12).

May we all keep the faith.

---

1 Naomi Wolf, *The Bodies of Others: The New Authoritarians*, COVID-19 and the *War Against the Human* (All Seasons Press, May 31, 2022), 307.

Chapter 2

The Same Persecution

Why was she whispering?

On a return visit to Romania a few years after my beloved father had passed away, I enjoyed a private, one-on-one talk with my mother. In this cherished mother-daughter conversation, Mom described how she was able to give birth to nine children during the days of communist rule. She told me how she and Dad were able to provide for all our needs despite the cruelties foisted on them by the dictatorial regime. But suddenly during our chat, my mother paused before lowering her voice to a whisper: "I did not tell this to anybody. When you and your brothers and sisters were little, your father was arrested by the communists. They put him in prison for six months because he dared to raise more chickens and sell more eggs to be able to make money to buy other things needed for all you children to be able to live."

How cruel is that? To lock up a father with small children at home and possibly let them starve because he took proactive steps to raise more chickens and provide for his family? I never heard that story as a child. Now as an adult with my own daughter, son-in-law, and three grandchildren, I see how hard they work to do anything necessary to provide food for their children and meet other needs. That makes me appreciate more deeply how my parents kept the persecutions of the communists a secret so we would not speak up and be persecuted as well for telling the truth.

Yet on that visit I wondered why she was whispering, more than two decades after the revolution that overthrew the dictator and expelled the communists from power? Because the oppression from communism programmed her mind in such a way that the effects lasted a lifetime. It made her lower her voice to the point of whispering in the same way we used to during the communists' reign, when we were censored and controlled for every word we spoke and every move we made.

Those who are too young to remember the sad state of the world under communist rule that originated in the Soviet Union and extended across Eastern Europe after World War II should never be deceived by the empty promises made by socialists and fellow travelers. The reality is that under the communist regimes in that part of the world, everything was tightly controlled. Namely, what you produced, what you bought or sold, what you ate, what you drank, what friends you had, and what you were thinking.

Many courageous believers who were brave enough to talk about God, share the gospel, and give Bibles to others lost their jobs; some were imprisoned for long periods of time and their families back home threatened. The secret police kept Christians under regular, ongoing surveillance. You couldn't have a private life.

The same thing goes on today in China. A few years ago the U.S. State Department issued a statement titled "China's Disregard for Human Rights." It said in part: "The government of the People's Republic of China (PRC), guided by a totalitarian ideology under the absolute rule of the Chinese Communist Party (CCP), deprives citizens of their rights on a sweeping scale and systematically curtails freedoms as a way to retain power. People in China cannot practice the religion or belief of their choice. They cannot express their opinions openly or form or join groups of their choosing without fear of harassment, arrest, or retribution. Members of minority groups are subject to mass arbitrary detention, Orwellian-style surveillance, political indoctrination, torture, forced abortions and sterilization, and state-sponsored forced labor." [2]

---

[2] "China's Disregard for Human Rights," U.S. Department of State, archived content from January 20, 2017 to January 20, 2021, https://2017-2021.state.gov/chinas-disregard-for-human-rights/, accessed October 29, 2024.

Lack of Freedom

During the communist rule in Romania, you could not own land or operate your own business. Christians were threatened, intimidated by the Securitate (one of the largest secret police forces in the Eastern bloc), and prohibited from owning or reading the Bible or Christian literature.

During my educational studies in Bucharest, I met a student from Zaire who came to study at the medical school in Romania. A strong believer filled with the Holy Spirit, she shared her experience with God in prayer in her country of origin. Her words moved me and prompted me to ask more about her spiritual life. One time she invited me to her dormitory for a time of prayer. Afterwards, the Securitate came and took me to the police station. They said I had committed a crime and threatened me with the loss of my job and the privilege of continuing my education.

Later, I invited my friend from Africa to visit my parents and grandparents in their village. The police showed up at my grandmother's home, confiscated our belongings, and took us to the police station. Claiming we were criminals, they held us for interrogations that lasted all day. Truthfully, we were guilty—of praying, singing, and worshiping God. We even recorded the songs that our sister from Zaire was singing with so much passion, praising God with all her heart. My parents and grandparents had never seen someone from Africa. They were delighted to meet someone from another continent with the same faith in Jesus Christ, and to see the power of the Holy Spirit working in people's hearts in a far-away place.

It was such a nice experience for the entire family and people from our church, but our enjoyment of that day was cut short. After a day-long investigation and intimidation in a frigid room at the station with no food or water, the police took us back to my parents' house. We remained under scrutiny for a long time after that.

Persecuted Again

Given this experience and the horrors of life under communism, I never imagined facing similar treatment in the USA. When the pandemic invaded our nation and neighbors in our adoptive home started getting deathly ill from the lethal pathogen that killed millions worldwide, I searched desperately for solutions. I started treating suffering patients, including some who were so sick they were facing a certain death sentence.

Little did I realize that my innate compassion for people that inspired me to offer early interventions that saved hundreds of lives would lead to endless investigations by the authorities. Specifically, the agency that regulates nurse practitioners (NP) and doctors of nursing practice (DNP). They exert authority over NPs and DNPs by determining who can hold a license to practice medicine. Without warning, I found my license stripped away by those whom I doubt treated a single patient infected by the deadly virus.

Without knowing it, I had embarked on a cause to not only save patients' lives, but also to battle for *truth and freedom* in medicine and stand against health care propaganda. And, against dictatorship, persecution, and communist-like tactics that are coming so quickly to the US, a free country built on Judeo-Christian principles by hard-working Americans. The health authorities stated that I had violated acceptable standards of care when I saved patients' lives! They insisted I had not followed "rules and regulations" as a primary care provider and DNP at the Good News Clinic. A clinic, by the way, which specializes in helping minorities, the homeless, the marginalized, and poor people who fall through the cracks. They couldn't afford insurance, nor did they qualify for social services. In short, they had no access to the health care system.

I volunteered my time during the early days of the pandemic, amid the fear, paranoia, and suspicion created by widespread lockdowns. I tirelessly treated and supported suffering patients desperate for help. I made myself available twenty-four hours a day to help people suffering as much from fear as the coronavirus. Then I heard the misguided attacks taking place against medical practitioners, doctors, and physicians with years of experience, who saved lives in the US and around the world.

Regardless of location, doctors and nurse practitioners with prescription privileges were banned from treating patients suffering with symptoms from the deadly virus. The reason? They used off-label meds that were safe and cost effective, for the purpose of saving lives. Yet a most strange development followed: if doctors prescribed an off-label medication for a Covid patient, many pharmacies refused to fill those prescriptions. In other words, the pharmacists at those drug stores were practicing medicine without a license. Because of the Orwellian oversight of government authorities, the pharmacists were afraid they would lose their license for filling those prescriptions. Yet the authority to prescribe and order medications for sick patients rests on physicians, not pharmacists.

This had never happened previously in the history of medicine. As a result, many patients went to primary care doctors and practitioners for treatment and wound up going home with no treatment. They were told to wait for their condition to deteriorate and their symptoms to get worse. This made the inflammation worse, leading to a "cytokine storm," which is a severe immune response where the body releases too many cytokines (cytokines are small proteins that act as messengers controlling the body's immune response) into the bloodstream too quickly. This cytokines storm, released by the immune system, was triggered by the spike protein from the Covid virus. It caused catastrophic damage in many patients' lungs, requiring hospitalization. Some needed intubation, which is when a tube is inserted into a patient's mouth to keep their airways open. Others needed mechanical ventilators. Many died prematurely.

Offering Compassion

As a health care and medical provider for more than thirty years, my skills had been sharpened by working with numerous patients, providing one-on-one care in many settings. This ranged from being a caregiver at the bedsides of patients with multiple chronic health conditions to those with severe disabilities (living in the same house for about twelve years and observing the progression of the person's condition to the end of their life). I had used a variety of medications for acute situations and for multiple chronic conditions. In addition, I worked in our memory care facilities for another thirteen years with patients suffering from Alzheimer's, dementia, and other kinds of infirmities and diseases.

I also worked as a clinician and primary care provider at Portland Adventist Community Services (PACS) and Good News free clinic, where seriously ill people sought care. By now, I had the knowledge, experience, and expertise, coupled with compassion for suffering patients, in my DNA. These experiences helped sharpen my clinical judgment and enabled me to make quick decisions regarding patient care. The years of training and experience in the health care field had paid dividends.

Given my background and help I had offered to the poor and downtrodden, the investigations launched against me for saving lives shocked me. Using my knowledge and expertise, I was confident that prescribing life-saving medications—even though they were off-label—was based on solid scientific evidence. And, such use included few or no side effects. Even the U.S. Food and Drug Administration's posting on off-label use of prescription medication says, "From the FDA perspective, once the FDA approves a drug, healthcare providers generally may prescribe the drug for an unapproved use when they judge that it is *medically appropriate for their patient*"[3] (emphasis added). Given this, I never dreamed of facing a Goliath-like battle.

Like me, many other frontline doctors had compassion to care for suffering patients during the pandemic, as Drs. Brian Tyson and

---

[3] "Understanding Unapproved Use of Approved Drugs 'Off Label,'" U.S. Food & Drug Administration, https://www.fda.gov/patients/learn-about-expanded-access-and-other-treatment-options/understanding-unapproved-use-approved-drugs-label, accessed October 29, 2024.

George Fareed chronicled in their 2022 book, Overcoming the COVID Darkness: How Two Doctors Successfully Treated 7000 Patients.

While health authorities frowned on the use of hydroxychloroquine, passionate doctors around the world treated suffering patients early in the disease process with this protocol. It did indeed prevent death and hospitalization, as the doctors wrote in their book. Among the examples they cited: Dr. Didier Raoult in France, who saved approximately 8,000 patients; Dr. Vipul Shas in India, 8,000 patients; Dr. Luigi Cavanna in Italy, 280 patients; senior clinical pharmacist Abdulrahman Mohana in Saudi Arabia, more than 2,700; Dr. Vladimir Zelenko (who died in 2022), around 3,000 patients; Dr. Heather Gessling, Columbia, Missouri's top-ranked family physician, who treated around 1,500 patients; and the authors successfully treating 7,000 patients. The cumulative total the authors reviewed came to approximately100,000 cases, with only thirty deaths, a 99.9 percent survival rate.[4]

These treatments generated worldwide news coverage. Take the story that appeared in Time magazine in April of 2020 about Dr. Cavanna's work in Italy. The head of the oncology ward at Piacenza hospital, he realized that too many seriously ill Covid patients were arriving in the emergency room "while most of them could have been treated at home earlier, before their symptoms became too grave.

"'When I realized that the emergency room was overcrowded with people already in serious condition, I knew something was wrong,' Cavanna explains. 'This is not a stroke or a heart attack, but a virus that can hit in different ways and that follows its course. We have to try to stop it before it damages the lungs in a way that is sometimes irreversible.' According to the data he collected during the first month, fewer than 10 (percent) of the patients he treated at home worsened to the point where they had to be hospitalized."[5]

---

4 Brian Tyson and George Fareed, Overcoming the COVID-19 Darkness: How Two Doctors Successfully Treated 7,000 Patients, (Independently published, 2022), 156.

5 Francesca Berardi, "The Italian Doctor Flattening the Curve by Treating COVID-19 Patients in Their Homes, Time, April 9, 2020, https://time.com/5816874/italy-coronavirus-patients-treating-home/.

Time also noted that until mid-April of 2020 he had been giving most of his patients hydroxychloroquine—commonly used for malaria and inflammatory disorders, such as rheumatoid arthritis—and an antiviral often prescribed for HIV. But after Italy's equivalent to the FDA issued an advisory to be careful in prescribing them together, Dr. Cavanna started using just hydroxychloroquine.

All these doctors and many others who treated early suffering patients with Covid symptoms saved their lives from premature death. Yet all endured the same hardship: being humiliated for their compassion in providing care to vulnerable people suffering from a deadly virus. They were threatened by medical establishments with the loss of their license and their career. They were censored and their character assassinated as they faced humiliation and persecution for the "crime" of saving lives. I ask: what is wrong with this picture?

Chapter 3

License Revoked

The medical director and staff at our small clinic were shocked when they learned my license had been revoked. The first to come to my rescue: Dr. Robert Sayson, a Harvard-educated physician who had traveled around the world on medical mission trips. In 2007, at the age of fifty-seven, he had walked away from a medical practice of fifteen years to open Good News Community Health Clinic. Located in the Portland suburb of Gresham, it had been a house, a pawn shop, and a tanning salon before Dr. Sayson purchased it. He and his wife also downsized their lifestyle and live off their savings so he can work fulltime for no salary.[6]

In asking the Oregon State Board of Nursing (OSBN) to reconsider its disciplinary action against me in April 2023 for allegedly "failing to take action to preserve client safety, failing to document client care information, and entering inaccurate documentation into a health record" (which were all false accusations), Dr. Sayson noted he based his appeal on the fact the disciplinary action invoked was disproportionate to the charges.

First, he pointed out that I had had a pristine record of caring for my patients, never had any prior complaint lodged against me with the board, and never had any malpractice cases charged against me in more than twenty of years as an OHSU-trained (Oregon Health & Science University) doctor of NP (nurse practitioner).

---

[6] "Dr. Bob Sayson founds Good News Community Health Center in Gresham to help needy," Oregon Live, January 27, 2012, ttps://www.oregonlive.com/gresham/2012/01/dr_bob_sayson_founds_good_news.html.

Among the alternatives he said the board could have taken: 1) a letter of reprimand or warning, 2) requiring enrollment in a continuing education course, 3) working under supervision, 4) paying a fine, 5) being placed under probation until alleged deficiencies were corrected, or 6) suspending my license until corrections are made. But, he said, the decision issued offered no recourse or opportunity to correct issues identified; it was permanent and irrevocable.

Dr. Sayson noted there was no crime committed, no harm done to a patient, no patient negligence, no patient complaints, no demonstration of a lack of continuing medical education or failure to consult with other specialists, no demonstration of employing harmful unscientific treatment protocols, no personal impairment of judgement or integrity, and no failure to document patient care and plans of treatment.

"She gave generous sacrificial service to our community during the pandemic, above and beyond the call of duty or personal safety concern," he wrote. "(This provided) timely needed treatment, resulting in great relief, prevention of hospitalization, and always with emotional, spiritual support with hope. The pandemic resulted in very limited health care availability and patients generally advised to 'sicken in place' before going to (an) emergency (department). No instructions or education to keep immune systems healthy or to prevent worsening of symptoms was offered to the community by usual places of health care, other than isolation."

Dr. Sayson reminded the board the American Nurses Association's code of ethics contains seven foundational principles: respect for autonomy (self-determination), beneficence (do good), non-maleficence (do no harm), justice (fairness), fidelity (keep promises), and veracity (tell the truth). Dr. Malos had upheld these foundational principles, he added, and gone beyond because of my compassion for suffering patients at a time of great uncertainty and fear. He also pointed out that the board's decision had hindered the clinic's ability to serve the community.

"On behalf of our community, we appeal to the honorable Board of Nursing who are firstly nurses, guided by the above mentioned ethical principles, to reconsider why Dr. Malos has been irrevocably and permanently barred from practicing as a well-trained (nurse practitioner) serving Oregonians," he concluded. "I believe that the honorable members of the Board of Nursing can wisely decide on a more equitable win-win solution that would allow Oregonians to continue to benefit from services provided at the Good News (clinic)."

Praying for Breakthrough

A strong believer who has practiced medicine for more than forty years, Dr. Sayson prays for every patient who allows him to do so, asking that God bring not only physical healing but also emotional and spiritual healing (which patients often need the most). I have had similar experiences, praying for patients during my practice while I volunteered more than fifteen thousand hours of service over two decades. With other dedicated volunteers, we provided care for those who were marginalized, homeless, poor, or needy immigrants. In short, "the least of these" Jesus spoke about in Matthew 25:40. People who had nobody to help them.

The OSBN did not investigate my sacrifices to provide care to the most vulnerable populations or try to discern the motivation behind my actions to treat suffering patients. Many of these victims had been left untreated and on the edge of the grave, with deteriorating and damaged lungs. As I mentioned in chapter 2, this deadly virus turned the immune system against itself, provoking a storm of cytokines and producing inflammation in the respiratory system. If not treated early enough to prevent hospitalization, this Covid-organized pneumonia could lead to premature death for many patients.

Experiencing Persecution

The board revoked my license for using a protocol developed by the best doctors, scientists, and experts with the greatest experience in medicine. It was based on the best scientific evidence available to alleviate pain and fear, making people feel better when they hurt badly, and preventing hospitalization and saving lives. Because of this treatment, people who might otherwise have died prematurely are alive today.

During this time of injustice and inhumane actions in the health field, I needed to run to the Word of God to strengthen myself. I suffered psychological trauma and great personal distress after they took away the joy of providing care for suffering patients. This was the highlight of my life, ever since I was a teenager in the village where I grew up and visited suffering families. Then I did not know anything about medicine, but I did know that if you feed the hungry, clothe the naked, and visit the sick you can help carry their burdens. This is one crucial reason that decades later I so love treating patients.

One time, I was meditating on the apostle Paul's letter (Philippians 1:12–14) and how he wrote that he needed to be put in prison so he could write more effectively and others would be encouraged to share their faith more boldly. For those persecuted for their faith, values, and beliefs, persecution is often the most valuable time of their spiritual lives. When under duress, they pray more effectively, write their stories, and share their experiences. During persecutions we must walk with God hand in hand, like the prophets who were not treated well when they were facing evil.

Dr. David Levy reaffirmed my observations when he encouraged me to write a book about my experiences. *The author of Gray Matter: A Neurosurgeon Discovers the Power of Prayer ... One Patient at a Time*[7] had faced persecution for his faith and for praying in Jesus's name, but did not give up. (You can imagine the hostility a professing believer would face on any modern college campus.) Once during a telephone conversation, he told me that the most the most powerful seasons of persecution, even during horrible injustice, are intended for our blessing. Even when we face bullying from ungodly people who are

---

[7] Tyndale House Publishers published this book in 2011.

anti-God and/or anti-Christ, we can get revelations and become more valuable to God's kingdom. Jesus Christ faced terrible injustice but His time on earth was His most valuable time of building God's Kingdom.

Dr. Levy added that during persecution, whether that described in the Bible or more recent times, God's children have suffered greatly. They have lost jobs, lost licenses, lost property, or were blamed, degraded, or demeaned. As he concluded our chat, he emphasized the truth of Philippians 3:10. Namely, that we can learn that knowing Christ and the power of His resurrection is not possible if we do not experience His sufferings, "that I may know Him and the power of His resurrection, and the fellowship of His sufferings, being conformed to His death."

During the communist regime in Romania and other Soviet bloc nations, Christians were deprived of their positions. How sad to see the same happen in a supposedly free nation. During the onset of the pandemic, Christians who had good jobs and enjoyed a good reputation for high morals and strong ethics were pushed out of those jobs for standing up for the truth. It is easy to get frustrated and angry at the injustice and inhumane actions when people were left to die. Yet, we know that anger is not healthy. Many people do not understand that bad attitudes and negative behavior can carry as much physical risk as untreated lethal pathogens.

Lost Compassion

During the early days of the pandemic, I saw firsthand in primary care health settings how doctors, nurses, and medical staff (the "healers") lost compassion for suffering people. This at a time when victims needed it the most. I saw videos of doors getting slammed in patients' faces, voices raised to those who were moving too slowly, or needed some oxygen or clean air to breathe, or who were scared by dictatorial attitudes displayed by receptionists or the folks who hid behind Plexiglas shields and wear-your-mask mandates. The tone of voice used by staff members in many clinics sickened me. I could hear the unkind hate behind "put your mask on" growls when there was no one else in that lobby. Instead of a soothing voice, harsh ones made many patients want to run away. Many patients were reluctant to return to a clinic or hospital for fear of facing more rejection, hatred, manipulation, dictatorial attitudes, or a lack of compassion and kindness.

Yet all this time, God was looking for people to stand in the gap for those who were suffering: "So I sought for a man among them who would make a wall, and stand in the gap before Me on behalf of the land, that I should not destroy it; but I found no one" (Ezek. 22:30, emphasis added). Regardless of the circumstances (and I realize the coronavirus frightened many people out of their wits) God always wants to see demonstrations of caring and compassion: "He has shown you, O man, what is good; and what does the Lord require of you but to do justly, to love mercy, and to walk humbly with your God?" (Mic. 6:8).

Given such words, it hurt me to see the lack of compassion for suffering patients in so many primary care settings. To me, it is unconscionable that people were told "there is no treatment for Covid" when in fact there were potential solutions. Because these remedies went against prevailing medical opinions (many proven later to be wrong or misguided), people were unable to access treatment for their symptoms. What a tragedy!

The Good Samaritan

Our emotions are affected by our faith. People of faith see things differently through God's eyes, unlike what many see with their physical eyes. When it came to suffering patients, my faith drove me to the place where I could not sit and do nothing. Reflecting about what Jesus would do in this situation if He saw people dying from all manner of diseases or if they were hungry and exhausted, I appreciated how He would be moved with compassion. He would be walking the streets, healing all and then feeding the multitudes because of His love for humanity.

The parable of the Good Samaritan (Luke 10:25–37) has moved people's heart for centuries. It prompted millions to search for ways to care for people. They built hospitals, erected tents, and provided other places to care for people who were sick or abandoned. During the early days of the pandemic, we were asked to abandon those who were suffering and unable to take care of themselves. Authorities told us to keep them in isolation and not treat early symptoms to reduce their suffering and prevent disaster in those families. We were to allow their symptoms to get worse until their lungs were destroyed by the virus's inflammatory process. Those who experienced breathing difficulties that lowered their oxygen and then went to emergency rooms (ER) were often turned back without treatment. As an example, my dear pastors went through this devastating and inhumane process, as they outline in the following letter:

> June 4, 2023
> To Whom It May Concern:
>
> We write to you as survivors of COVID-19, Delta variant, July 2021. We are both septuagenarians and otherwise healthy up to that date. Both of us contracted this virus, five days apart, and suffered near-death symptoms. Low oxygenation levels (85 percent), fatigue and malaise contributed to an inability to concentrate and to make correct decisions.
>
> It was the intervention of a nurse friend and (Mrs.) Rodica Malos who cared for our every need. As you recall, no physician's office took in-person appointments. Ambulances were called on five occasions between the two of us and due to the critical shortage of hospital beds, we were unsuccessful in acquiring acute care. It was the intervention of (Mrs.) Malos, who saw us via FaceTime (and) fielded calls from our nurse caregiver, and ordered life-saving in-home oxygen therapy that saved our lives. The prescribed scientific protocols were followed and we believe helped maintain us until we were

finally admitted to ICUs. The symptoms were abated by prompt pharmaceutical and medical protocols, proven by other practitioners worldwide. We owe our lives to Rodica Malos and to the prescriptions/treatments received.

Sincerely,
Pastor __________
Pastor __________

As a primary care provider, I found it unthinkable that medical authorities forced us to disengage from patients. We couldn't even ask questions about why we could not treat symptoms from the inflammatory process that caused multiple complications in the human body. We couldn't treat patients the same way we had done (in my case) for thirty-plus years, even when patients improved when we prescribed off-label medications, preventing further damage or hospitalization.

The accusers from the state nursing board wanted to know why I had prescribed budesonide via nebulizer for patients (among its many uses, budesonide can treat mild to moderate Crohn's disease, an inflammatory bowel disease). I did this when patients' oxygen level started to drop below 94 percent due to the inflammatory process in the lungs. This caused damage and put the patients at risk of developing Covid pneumonia. And, many scientific studies had shown that budesonide reduced inflammation in the lungs, thus saving lives.

One example is a June 14, 2022 article in the Journal of the American Medical Association by Dr. William E. Cayley Jr. He noted that "in antiviral medications, it is important to mention that 2 studies published last year demonstrated the clinical utility of inhaled budesonide for outpatient treatment of COVID-19. In the STOIC trial of 146 adults with early COVID-19 who were rando-mized to receive inhaled high-dose budesonide vs usual care, budesonide reduced the primary outcome (urgent care visits, emergency department visits, or hospitalization) with a number needed to treat of 8 and shortened the time to clinical recovery by 1 day.

"In the PRINCIPLE trial of 4700 older patients with COVID-19 who were randomized to receive usual care vs inhaled high-dose budesonide vs. other treatments, budesonide reduced the time to first self-reported recovery by almost 3 days compared with usual care. In the quest to develop, distribute, and utilize therapeutics for COVID-19, it important not to overlook the demonstrated benefit of a medication that is already in current use and is relatively easily accessible."[8]

I saw this with my treatment of patients who took budesonide. It reduced their inflammation and they felt better immediately. This is in stark contrast to those who received no treatment and their symptoms grew much worse.

One example of the positive effects of budesonide is an eighty-nine-year-old patient's blood oxygen level, which improved from 91 percent to 95 percent after twenty minutes of the drug, administered via a nebulizer. When I went to visit her at her home to assist with treatment, she was weak and lethargic from the damage done by coronavirus. The nursing board investigator accused me of visiting patients in their home and endangering them when they were in isolation. I cried when I heard that accusation, knowing I had helped save neighbors' lives—like that of this eighty-nine-year-old woman—preventing further suffering and unnecessary, premature death.

The Need to Stand

Many doctors recognize the need to stand for the truth and freedom. They are like the Old Testament prophet, Jeremiah, who wrote, "But if I say, 'I will not mention his word or speak anymore in his name,' his word is in my heart like a fire, a fire shut up in my bones. I am weary of holding it in; indeed, I cannot" (Jer. 20:9 NIV).

[8] William E. Cayley Jr., MD, "COVID-19 Treatments for Nonhospitalized Patients," *Journal of the American Medical Association*, June 14, 2022, https://jamanetwork.com/journals/jama/article-abstract/2793260.

Indeed, the Word of God led me to have courage to stand up for the truth and offer compassion for suffering people, a desire He instilled in my heart. It felt like that fire shut up in my bones described by Jeremiah. The Word helped point me in the right direction, even if I was going against the grain and opposing the established medical authorities. I vowed to make the right decision and help people when they needed it the most.

Our good deeds have eternal values. Paul addressed that in his letter to the Romans, when he said that God "'will render to each one according to his deeds': eternal life to those who by patient continuance in doing good seek for glory, honor, and immortality; but to those who are self-seeking and do not obey the truth, but obey unrighteousness—indignation and wrath, tribulation and anguish" (Rom. 2:6–9, emphasis added).

We need to do good deeds, even when it will bring retribution.

Chapter 4

Shocking Development

As mentioned earlier, the revocation of my medical license was a devastating development. As this reality sank in, I realized that when it came to evaluating health care decisions and reaching reasonable judgments, my thoughts and approach no longer mattered. The freedom to think freely had been snatched away. The medical establishment and state nursing board placed restrictions on my critical thinking skills and clinical judgments as a general practitioner. My education and experience were deemed irrelevant. Everything I learned in more than ten years of classroom, clinical, and hospital settings? Poof. Intensive continuing education of a hundred hours every two years? Didn't matter. Nor did my experience in providing direct care of people as a caregiver and time as a registered nurse (in my own adult foster care homes/memory care facilities).

More than twenty years of experience as a nurse practitioner and doctor of nursing practice also seemed to make no difference. Not only had I spent hour upon hour at the bedsides of dying patients, I held many of their hands as they slipped out of consciousness. I had practiced general medicine as a primary care provider, taking care of extremely sick people. They included immigrants, minorities, the marginalized, homeless, and impoverished (some were so poor they didn't have five dollars for needed medication).

The nursing board's accusations were based in criticism for using my critical thinking skills and judgments, based on years of training at one of the nation's most prestigious universities.

A protocol that saved countless lives but was banned in health care settings during the pandemic is illustrated in the following chart.

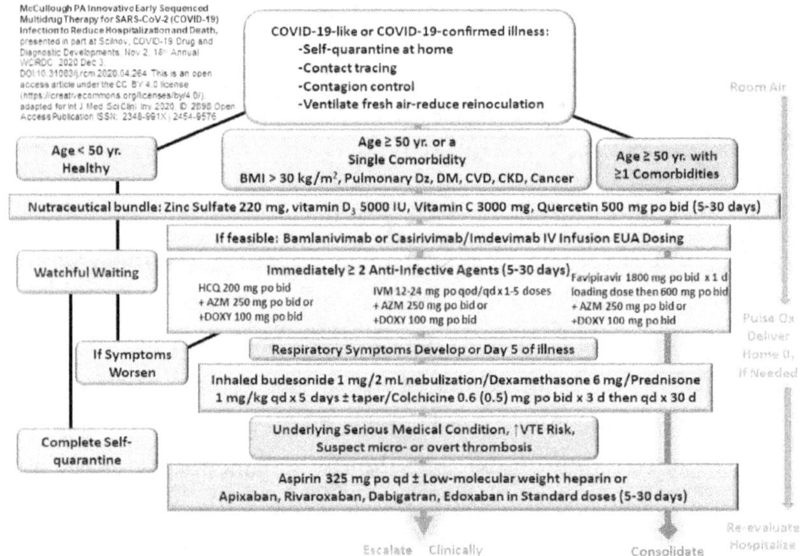

The protocol presented above contains medications that I had used for patients with multiple chronic conditions for many years. Any doctor, general practitioner, or specialist of any kind is familiar with those medications; they know they are safe when used for short-term treatment of symptoms similar to those of COVID-19. The results of various tests using these medicals are well-documented in scientific literature.

The therapeutic response diagram that follows shows the window of time for early treatment is the ambulatory phase during the first seven days. Such action in that time frame can save patients' lives. The earlier the treatments are administered, the more effective the results.

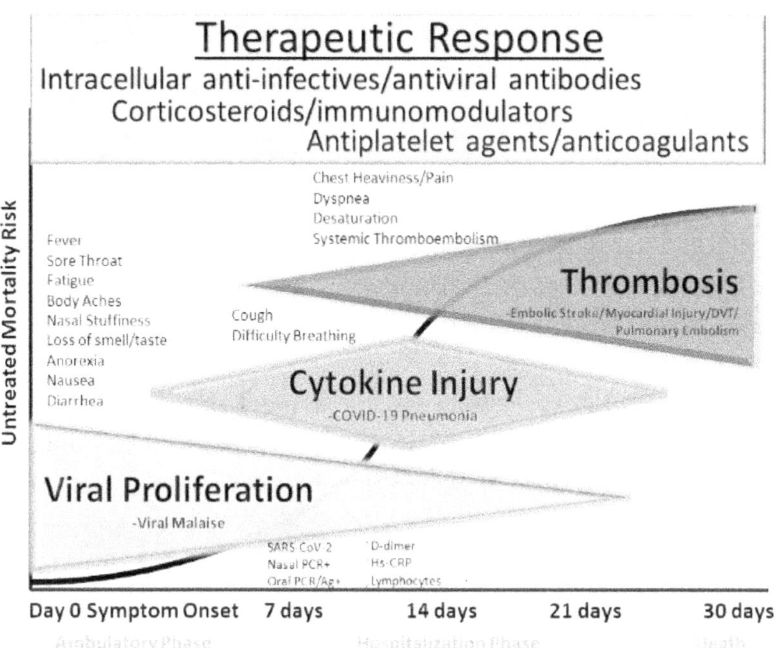

A Spiritual Battle

As a Christian with a strong background in faith, I believe we are facing a spiritual war—an outrageous battle with evil spirits, manifested physically in our nation's health care system. Never in my life have I seen this kind of psychological and physical war against humanity. It chills me when I reflect on the fact that medical providers let people with serious symptoms suffer while doing little to make them better or prevent damage to their vital organs. Denying people early treatment left them susceptible to premature death. It disturbed me to watch news media reports closely and see no one talking about health promotion and disease-prevention any longer.

Since I had spent my entire academic life studying health promotion and disease-prevention, I realized that someone should take action to promote physical, emotional, and spiritual health, since all have an eternal impact. During the pandemic I did not have the peace to "do nothing" and let patients sit with a deadly virus while their symptoms grew worse. Not when I knew there were safe medications that could reduce the viral load and inflammatory process that could destroy people's vital organs.

In health care, physicians know that inflammation is the mother of all diseases. But awareness of these medicines was suppressed at the federal and state government levels, as well as by mass media and other authorities, from top medical leaders to local pharmacies. Suffering people had to endure a disease process that could have been treated early with minimum damage.

I am still in shock over such action and the consequences to suffering people. I am appalled that no one has been held responsible for the gross negligence in the health field during the pandemic. It is outrageous how those in power suppressed early interventions and silenced doctors who tried to take action to speak the truth and fight for patients' lives.

Many doctors who stood against the tyranny were censored or threatened with the loss of their medical license, career, and profession. They lived with fear gripping their heart, soul, and spirit. Fortunately, there were many doctors who were bold and climbed out of their comfort zone to alert the world, including at the international level, and wake up the medical community to the injustices done to suffering people.

The Impact of Fear

Though a divine appointment, I received an invitation to speak at the International Covid Summit, ICS-4, at the Romanian Parliament in Bucharest in November of 2023 (I will go into more background about ICS in the next chapter). I spoke about the fear spread during the pandemic—and the consequences of instilling fear in people's mind through propaganda, lies, and dictatorship. Here is a shortened version of my talk; this may give a sense of my inner pain and psychological distress at the time.

Warm welcome to doctors, scientists, and experts of the world—the "giants of medicine"—to the city of Bucharest, the capital of Romania, the most beautiful city in the world (and my hometown for eighteen years before I fled to the USA to escape the lies and oppression of communism). I thank you from the bottom of my heart for being willing to share from your knowledge, experience, and expertise so millions of lives around the world have been saved, including mine. Like my patients told me many times: "We owe you our lives" when I treated them for symptoms from a deadly virus, I want to tell you the same. I owe you my life. And on behalf of the Romanian communities in the Portland (Oregon) and Vancouver (Washington) areas in the USA who were saved through early interventions per protocol developed by top experts (and some of them are here in this room), I thank you.

The pandemic's devastating catastrophes led to fear due to:

- Prohibited early treatment for a deadly virus COVID-19 "sicken-in-place" and "hospital-dependent" approach that led to premature death. Many are still grieving for their loved ones, who died unnecessarily.
- Imposed evil lockdown of the world and economy that destroyed peoples' lives.
- Destroyed small businesses and middle class's wellbeing and their families.
- Closed churches, places of spiritual and emotional healing, when needed the most.
- Made people distance from each other and to isolate, leading to mental health crisis.
- Deprived from medical, mental, emotional, and spiritual support during crisis.
- Mask mandates not effective, but dangerous when used for prolonged hours unnecessarily, due to inhaling back own CO2 and microbes from the mouth.
- Exaggerated death count to frighten and scare population.

- Hidden adverse effects of the COVID-19 mRNA vaccines "gene therapy" from the public.
- Mandating experimental "vaccine/gene therapy" that turns the body against itself.
- Doctors and nurses lost jobs due to mandates creating shortages and chaos in health care during the pandemic.
- Doctors and nurses lost licenses and careers for saving lives with early interventions.

A study titled "The Implications of COVID-19 for Mental Health and Substance Use"[9] published on March 20, 2023 demonstrated that the pandemic has affected the public's mental health and well-being in a variety of ways, including isolation, loneliness, job loss, financial instability, illness, and grief. In the same study were reported job losses of 52.8 percent, excessive drinking increased[10] and alcohol-induced death rates increased by 38 percent, an increase in substance abuse[11] [12] drug overdose death rate rose by 50 percent, youth mental health (problems) further increased, a recent uptick in gun violence, and negative impact on child's mental health, showing that Covid pandemic time was also "a mind virus."

Fear and Stress

Science journalist Mary Van Beusekom stated that COVID-19 has tripled the rate of depression in US adults in all demographic groups—especially in those with financial worries—and the rise is much higher than after previous major traumatic events, according to a study

---

[9] Nirmita Panchal, Heather Sanders, Robin Rudowitz, and Cynthia Cox, KFF (independent nonprofit providing health policy research, polling, and news), March 20, 2023, https://www.kff.org/mental-health/issue-brief/the-implications-of-covid-19-for-mental-health-and-substance-use/

[10] "Effect of increased alcohol consumption during COVID-19 pandemic on alcohol-associated liver disease: A modeling study, Hepatology, Volume 75, Issue 6, 1480-1490, December 8, 2021, https://aasldpubs.onlinelibrary.wiley.com/doi/abs/10.1002/hep.32272.

[11] Amanda Roberts, Jim Rogers, Rachel Mason, Aloysius Niroshan Siriwardena, Todd Hogue, Gregory Adam Whitley, and Graham R. Law, "Alcohol and other substance abuse during the COVID-19 pandemic: A systematic review, Drug and Alcohol Dependence, October 29, 2021, https://pmc.ncbi.nlm.nih.gov/articles/PMC8559994/.

[12] Nirmita Panchal, Heather Sanders, Robin Rudowitz, and Cynthia Cox, "Substance Use Issues Are Worsening Alongside Access to Care," KFF, August 12, 2021, https://www.kff.org/policy-watch/substance-use-issues-are-worsening-alongside-access-to-care/.

published yesterday on the JAMA (Journal of the American Medical Association) Network Open.[13] The fear of dying from an "invisible enemy" cripples people. Increased anxiety and depression have been noticed since COVID-19 started. Authors Mark Czeisler, Rashon Lane, Emiko Petrosky, and others demonstrated that "the coronavirus disease 2019 (COVID-19) pandemic has been associated with mental health challenges related to the morbidity and mortality caused by the disease and to mitigation activities, including the impact of physical distancing and stay-at-home orders. Symptoms of anxiety disorder and depressive disorder increased considerably in the United States during June of 2020, compared with the same period in 2019."[14]

The battle with incertitude and unpredictability continues even today in managing this "invisible enemy" and the struggles continue in proving what works and what does not work, scientifically, in the absence of scientific results of randomized clinical studies. Many patients stated that they went through the "valley of the shadow of death." One particular patient, R (dear to our family), confesses: "I have seen death last night with my own eyes" when symptoms from COVID-19 got worse at home without early intervention from primary care practitioners. We knew from the past that "75–90 (percent) of doctor visits are related to stress," according to Dr. Joseph Goldberg, MD.[15] Various studies estimate that stress costs American industry more than $300 billion annually. That alone affects the economy, leading to more stress increases and more diseases. I believe with no doubt that increased exponentially from fear during the pandemic.

Fear is the greatest enemy of our health: physically, mentally, and spiritually.

---

[13] Catherine K. Ettman, BA; Salma M. Abdalla, MD, MPH; Gregory H. Cohen, MPhil, MSW, PhD; Laura Sampson, PhD; Patrick M. Vivier, MD, PhD; Sandro Galea, MD, DrPH; "Prevalence of Depression Symptoms in US Adults Before and During the COVID-19 Pandemic," JAMA Network Open, September 2, 2020; htps://jamanetwork.com/journals/jamanetworkopen/fullarticle/2770146.

[14] Mark E. Czeisler; Rashon I. Lane, MA; Emiko Petrosky, MD; et. al., "Mental Health, Substance Abuse, and Suicidal Ideation During the COVID-19 Pandemic – United States, June 24-30, 2020," Centers for Disease Control, August 14, 2020, https://www.cdc.gov/mmwr/volumes/69/wr/mm6932a1.htm.

[15] Joseph F. Goldberg, M.D., https://www.josephgoldbergmd.com/, accessed November 5, 2024.

Fear of COVID-19 was (and still) is overwhelming and extremely stressful for everybody, instilling fear in people's minds and spirits that will lead to anxiety and sadness. Fear causes a shift in neurotransmitters and neurochemicals that are released in our body while serotonin, dopamine, melatonin, and other neurochemical levels decrease and further cause depression. The neurotransmitters imbalance may cause lack of sleep, leading to sleep deprivation weakening the immune system, thus increasing susceptibility to more illness.

Other Impacts

Fear affects people's brains and the immune system. Fear triggers thoughts and emotions that send signals to the hypothalamus that sends messages to the pituitary gland. This starts secreting adrenocorticotropic hormones, stimulating the adrenal gland to release cortisol and epinephrine. High cortisol level suppresses the immune system, which then becomes ineffective in fighting against viruses. Fear increases the chances of getting the virus by lowering the immune system that fights COVID-19. (Dr. David Levy, MD, the best neurosurgeon in the world, talks about this in his video, "Fear in Crisis - Part 1, Help for Coronavirus COVID-19, Overcoming Anxiety").[16]

Dr. Frank Jenkins and two other researchers have noted that "psychological stress, acting through *increased levels of catecholamine and/or cortisol, can increase DNA damage* and/or reduce repair mechanisms, resulting in increased risk of DNA mutations leading to carcinogenesis."[17]

The pandemic's effects can last for generations through epigenetics. In other words, genetic changes from fear and stress during the pandemic can be passed down through gene expression,

[16] You can see this video at https://www.youtube.com/watch?v=nfrbm1dvZal.

[17] Frank J. Jenkins, Bennett Van Houten, Dana H. Bovbjerg, "Effects on DNA Damage and/or Repair Processes as Biological Mechanisms Linking Psychological Stress to Cancer Risk," Journal of Applied Biobehavioral Research, 2014 March 4;19(1):3-23, https://pmc.ncbi.nlm.nih.gov/articles/PMC4039216/, emphasis added.

affecting the next generations. Mother's memories (and associated emotional thoughts) will be transmitted to the next generation, even in utero, through gene expression. Every person's life starts with one DNA at conception. Fear affects trillions of cells, including mitochondria, the "electric panel" of the cell. They are affected by low oxygen levels, caused by injuries from the inflammatory process due to the virus and vaccines for COVID-19 and from fear and stress in every vital organ.

High levels of fear and stress also lead to unhealthy decisions, behaviors, and practices, with their subsequent degenerative diseases as: heart disease, musculoskeletal diseases, neurological deficits, lung disease, infections, gastrointestinal distress, degenerative disease, metabolic syndrome, autoimmune diseases, mental disorders, cancer, and psychological distress.

Yet, fear and stress could have been alleviated through early treatment for COVID-19 symptoms. We know that love casts out fear, even in medicine. John put it best when he wrote, "There is no fear in love; but perfect love casts out fear, because fear involves torment. But he who fears has not been made perfect in love" (1 John 4:18).

One of my patients who was struggling with COVID-19 asked, "Why in the primary care setting are general practitioners and providers so relaxed and not prescribing medications to treat patients with COVID-19 symptoms at home?" I asked myself the same question: "Why am I relaxed in primary care, doing nothing for our suffering patients with coronavirus? If I do not treat them, they will die."

Preventing Hospitalization

The "sicken-in-place" and "hospital-dependent" policies were not the right approach. Early intervention was a solution of choosing life. As God told Moses: "I call heaven and earth as witnesses today against you, that I have set before you life and death, blessing and cursing; therefore choose life, that both you and your descendants may live" (Deut. 30:19).

In a 2021 article for the American Journal of Medicine, Dr. Peter McCullough and a team of other physicians stated that "therapeutic approaches based on these principles include 1) reduction of reinoculation, 2) combination antiviral therapy, 3) immune-modulation, 4) antiplatelet/antithrombotic therapy, and 5) administration of oxygen, monitoring, and telemedicine."[18] I consider that God gave humanity gifts as science and faith to save people's lives from a deadly virus.

Dr. Vladimir Zelenko treated thousands of patients suffering from symptoms from COVID-19 in the New York area with a protocol that saved lives. It included:

- Fundamental principles. Treat patients based on clinical suspicion as soon as possible, preferably within the first five days of symptoms. Perform PCR testing, but do not withhold treatment pending results.
- Risk-stratify patients. Low risk: those below age sixty, no comorbidities, and clinically stable. High risk: Those older than sixty or younger but with comorbidities, or clinically unstable.
- Treatment options.
- Low risk: over-the-counter options:
  1. Elemental zinc, 50 mg. once daily for seven days.
  2. Quercetin, 500 mg. twice a day for seven days or epigallocatechin-gallate (EGCG) 400 mg. once a day for seven days.
  3. Vitamin C, 1000 mg. once a day for seven days.
  4. Rest, oral fluids, and close follow-up with doctor.

- High risk patients.
  1. Elemental zinc, 50 mg. once a day for seven days.

[18] Peter A. McCullough, MD, et. al., "Pathophysiological Basis and Rationale for Early Outpatient Treatment of SARS-CoV-2 (COVID-19) Infection, The American Journal of Medicine, Volume 134, Issue 1, 16-22, January 2021, https://www.amjmed.com/article/S0002-9343(20)30673-2/full.

2. Hydroxychloroquine (HCQ) 200 mg. two times a day for seven days. If HCQ not available, quercetin 500 mg. three times a day for seven days or EGCG, 400 mg. two times a day for seven days.
3. Azithromycin, 500 mg. once a day for five days or doxycycline, 100 mg. two times a day for seven days.
4. Vitamin C, 1000 mg. once a day for seven days.
5. Rest, oral fluids, and close follow-up with doctor.

Additional treatment options should be uniquely custom tailored for every patient, but may include:

1. Ivermectin, 6 mg. two times a day for one week.
2. Budesonide, 1 mg./2 cc. solution via nebulizer two times a day for seven days.
3. Dexamethasone, 6 mg. one time a day for seven days.
4. Blood thinners (i.e. Lovenox).
5. Home oxygen.
6. Home IV fluids.

Note: If possible, keep patients out of the hospital.

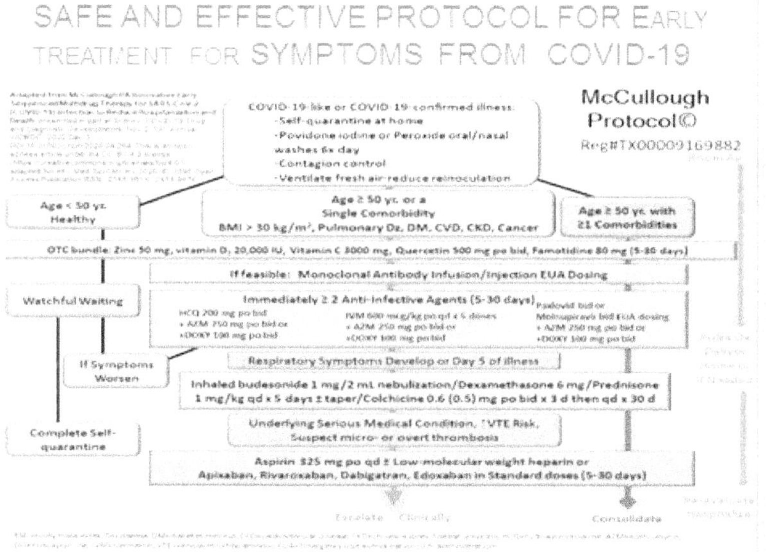

This protocol was included in the previously-mentioned article in the The American Journal of Medicine, but the information about the algorithm was not disseminated. Because it was suppressed by authorities at every level, we had to struggle with a lack of guidance, no solutions, and unnecessary premature deaths. I consider that gross negligence in our health care system—the greatest failure of medicine in the twenty-first century. This should never happen again.

Treatment must start in the first three to five days of exposure to coronavirus. If early treatment is banned, the cytokines storm causes injuries due to the inflammatory process, leading to hospitalization. If prophylactic treatment is not initiated early, then thrombosis, embolism, stroke, myocardial injuries, and pulmonary embolism are the results.

I honor and applaud Dr. Peter McCullough and all the experts for the hard work to save lives with their protocol (including Dr. Zelenko, who is watching from heaven and smiling). More and more studies are showing good results when HCQ is used early.

In addition, my experience in treating patients with ivermectin was absolutely amazing. One of the patients who experienced advanced symptoms from COVID-19 and whose oxygen levels dropped below 88 percent at night was extremely weak, tired, and desperate for medical care. She refused to go to the emergency room because of her fear of hospitalization. It was too late to start HCQ, but she followed the protocol mentioned above, and I added ivermectin for three days.

The patient's oxygen levels increased from 88 percent to 93 percent after the first dose in less than twenty-four hours, to 95 percent after the second dose, and to 97 percent after the third dose. The patient recovered and was happy that these medications were available. My heart is full of thanks to God and those prominent physicians, general practitioners, and specialists who advocated for the most vulnerable populations during COVID-19.

Other Remedies

A healthy lifestyle with a healthy diet, including fresh fruits and vegetables, and regular exercise, will also reduce inflammation in the body. It will improve the immune system, which helps fight viral and bacterial infections and repair the vital organs from damages done by the spike proteins from both the virus and the vaccine.

Emotional and spiritual needs are real and must be addressed to reduce stress from fear, anxiety, and depression. As I like to say, prayer is medicine. Meditation through prayer is the best way to cope with stress. Scientific literature has documented prayer's healthy impact on the brain. It reduces stress; lowers cortisol levels produced by high levels of stress; decreases anxiety; prevents panic attacks, depression, and bad behavior; corrects unhealthy emotions; reduces pain; lowers blood pressure; promotes rapid healing; and prevents infection.

Neuroscientists have discovered that the frontal lobe can shrink with aging, causing Alzheimer's disease, but prayer stimulates the frontal lobe and prevents shrinkage! Prayer is an antiaging exercise that causes new neurons to develop when you meditate in prayer. Prayer will calm an overactive brain, reduce anxiety, and promote healthy growth in children. Many doctors are praying for their patients' physical and spiritual health.

Proposal based on the science—evidence in scientific literature to prevent catastrophes again:

- Outpatient early treatment protocol for symptomatic COVID-19 infections
- Early diagnosis and early treatment (first three to five days)
- Massive education about disease process of COVID-19
- Establish community clinics for public access to early treatment of symptomatic COVID-19 infections
- Do not lock down public schools, businesses, places of worship, and other facilities

- High-risk health workers, high-risk teachers, and nursing home patients should take prophylaxis, especially during periods when there are high case numbers

We need a massive educational effort about early symptoms and early interventions to save lives, especially since regular Covid flare-ups have occurred in recent times. Patients must know the acceptable numbers for blood pressure, heart rate, respiration rate, temperature, blood sugar, and oxygen saturation, and start treatment in the first week of contacting the virus. But avoid lapsing into fretting and worry. As Paul wrote, "For God hath not given us the spirit of fear; but of power, and of love, and of a sound mind" (2 Tim. 1:7 KJV).

A few other worthwhile thoughts:

- "Whoever saves a single life is considered by scripture to have saved the whole world." (Sanhedrin 37a, the Talmud).[19]
- Faith is the antidote for fear: "And He has on His robe and on His thigh a name written: KING OF KINGS AND LORD OF LORDS" (Rev. 19:16).
- The power NOT to fear is in us.
- "For I am not ashamed of the gospel of Christ, for it is the power of God to salvation for everyone who believes, for the Jew first and also for the Greek" (Rom. 1:16).

---

[19] Rabbi Dan Moskovitz, Temple Shalom, Vancouver, BC, "Save One Life, Save the Entire World (Including Yourself)," Religious Action Center, May 24, 2019, https://rac.org/blog/save-one-life-save-entire-world-including-yourself.

Chapter 5

Divine Appointments

While I have written three books[20] and worked in the health care field in many roles in the US for more than three decades, I spent all my time in medical or Christian circles. So if anyone asks how I wound up attending the Conservative Political Action Conference in February of 2024, I explain that it happened because of a divine appointment.

In my desperate search for justice after the Oregon nursing board revoked my nurse practitioner's license—the license that allowed me to practice general medicine independently as a primary care provider for more than two decades—I learned about America's Frontline Doctors (AFLD) holding a White Coat Summit in front of the Supreme Court in July of 2023 and decided to attend.

What I learned about Frontline Doctors is they were in reality dedicated physicians who were persecuted for telling the truth, fighting for freedom, and saving lives. Through a divine appointment I received an invitation to attend this meeting. When I joined the doctors, scientists, and medical practitioners who were dedicated to speaking the truth about early treatment to save lives, it changed my perspective on life. And, sharing about the catastrophes that occurred during the pandemic due to the gross negligence in clinical practices, flimsy mask mandates, social distancing, and lockdowns of businesses, churches, and schools. What really stirred the hornet's nest was them

---

[20] The first was titled *Find Your Peace: Supernatural Solutions Beyond Science for Fear, Anxiety, and Depression*. It was published by Siloam, an imprint of Charisma House, in February of 2020. Two others were released the following year by Triology Christian Publishing.

describing the damage done by the medical community and government's propaganda and censorship.

The morning of the press conference in front of the Supreme Court, many of us were waiting in the lobby of a Washington, DC hotel for a shuttle bus. Some doctors were busily reconnecting with old acquaintances, while others checked their emails or text messages. I moved around trying to find a chair to sit in while we waited, although many seemed content to stand.

A "Chance" Meeting

As I stood on the left side of the spacious lobby, checking my messages, I raised my eyes. On my right side I saw a man who was also checking his messages. At first I thought he might be an angel, but in reality he was the renowned Dr. Robert W. Malone. If you haven't heard of him, Dr. Malone is a physician, inventor, scientist, speaker, bioethicist, journalist, and author.[21] I did not know how he wound up standing next to me. I had seen him on television several times on news broadcasts (even in Romania), but never in person or so close. Thoughts surged through my mind; I did not know what to do. Should I say something? Or turn to the left and walk away, pretending that I did not see him? After all, I am a rather shy person and ordinarily do not talk to strangers.

Still, he wasn't really a stranger, since I had seen him on TV, as well as at many of his public speeches or presentations. I knew what he stood for in medicine and political life. As I debated with myself internally (how do I behave around a genius with such a brilliant mind?) I heard myself say, "I saw you on the TV news in Romania." While his eyes were trained on his phone, reading, he suddenly raised his eyes when he heard my strong Romanian accent.

"I saw you on Romanian TV news," I repeated.

---

[21] His latest book, *PsyWar,* released in October of 2024. Coauthored with his wife, Jill, the 416-page book is subtitled "Enforcing the New World Order." It exposes the history and tactics of modern psychological warfare on the American people and suggests ways citizens can resist totalitarian control.

Smiling, he replied that he had been invited to the third International Covid Summit (ICS) event. ICS started as a grassroots movement by a small group of doctors and others who wanted answers to many questions and contradictory information that surfaced soon after the start of the pandemic. This questioning of the popular narrative spurred further action and created an international community dedicated to pushing for open inquiries and the pursuit of the truth.

At ICS-3 Dr. Malone had met with a Member of the European Parliament (MEP) from Romania, Cristian Terhes. The ICS organizers had arranged another summit in Bucharest in the Parliament building that November; Dr. Malone said I should participate in that session. Adrenaline surged through my body to receive that kind of invitation from such a giant in the medical field. Thoughts from the past rushed through my mind, especially memories of the communist regime when I lived in Bucharest.

I remember vividly watching Nicolae Ceausescu's minions constructing the huge Parliament building—internationally, second in size only to the Pentagon. It overwhelmed me with joy to think that the same building erected by dictators, oppressors, tyrants, and suppressors of the truth would now resound with the voices of people standing up for the truth and fighting for freedom. It also filled me with joy when Dr. Malone connected me with his team in that moment by having them text me all the necessary details about the event (after all, friends will share such information).

I felt in my spirit a great peace as God again proved His power through the Holy Spirit. As His Word promises, He will ordain our steps so we are at the right place at the right time at the right moment. Psalm 37:23–24 says, "The steps of a man are established by the LORD, when he delights in his way; though he fall, he shall not be cast headlong, for the LORD upholds his hand" (ESV).

Healing Begins

This is why I say there are no "chance" meetings or coincidences, only divine appointments. After all, Dr. Malone knew nothing about me. I traveled to Washington, DC that summer with a broken heart over being persecuted by Oregon's medical establishment. I had been attacked for saving hundreds of lives during the pandemic, and while volunteering much of my time. That included being on call 24/7. I gave a piece of my heart to every suffering patient, many who had been condemned to die. I sacrificed my profession and my license to save their lives.

During that moment in the hotel lobby, I felt the healing process begin. That's how I developed a deeper appreciation for unspeakable joy as a sure antidote for sadness and depression. I already knew that joy released dopamine, endorphins, and other neurotransmitters to help bring healing of my emotions from a broken heart and physical healing for my body, which had been negatively affected by the tyranny of those in authority. And yet, this was a deeper, profound supernatural moment; the joy of the Lord became my strength that day. An exhilaration filled me from head to toe, in a way that surpassed human reasoning or understanding.

For me to participate at the International Covid Summit ICS-4 in Bucharest was huge. Even to speak at the Parliament ... it was almost impossible for me to believe. Living under that cruel regime, I had suffered in great poverty my eighteen years in Burcharest; so did two million others living in the metropolitan area. After watching that building rising up under Ceausescu's dictatorship, I dearly loved having the opportunity to be on the same stage about three decades later, speaking about truth and freedom. This is why I will never forget the divine appointment in Washington that led to my talk in Bucharest. Then from that unbelievable event, I received the invitation from ICS leaders to attend the CPAC the following year, which led me to write the book you hold in your hands (or read on your computer or smartphone).

AMERICA'S FRONTLINE DOCTORS STANDING UP FOR THE TRUTH AT ANY COST

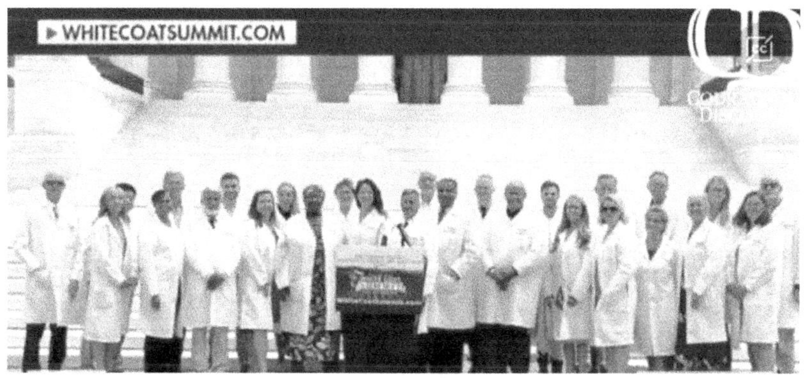

That July day in 2023, as the press conference began, various members of Frontline Doctors spoke in urgent tones. They appealed to millions of potential listeners to hear the heart of these superheroes who were not afraid to stand up for the truth and fight for freedom. Dr. Stella Immanuel issued a call to America to wake up and return to God, as well as recognizing the dangerous path the nation was on toward dictatorship, totalitarianism, and tyranny. Others echoed her words, insisting we must stand for truth and freedom or lose it.

I felt it in my bones: America was on the edge of losing the freedom to live. I admired these doctors for their willingness to withstand the ridicule and loss of their professional reputation and standing in the medical community for speaking out against the suffocation of tyranny in the nation's health care system. They were calling for the necessity of letting America live and not snuff out our cherished freedoms. Their voices echoed in my ears a year after that unique experience and will continue to reverberate for years to come. My eyes filled with tears as I remembered the heartache, oppression, and tyranny of living for more than thirty years in an absolute dictatorship.

Dr. Immanuel is the medical doctor who wrote more than 100,000 prescriptions for patients suffering from Covid, including me.

I quickly became her patient after my own doctor refused to treat me when I was suffering from symptoms of Covid and my blood oxygen level started to drop. My primary care provider in Oregon insisted "there is no treatment for Covid" at the very time I needed treatment the most. But Dr. Immanuel treated me via telehealth with effective medications. In three to four days I felt much better. She saved my life and is my hero.

Ironically, Dr. Immanuel was threatened, humiliated, and faced false charges from mainstream media. That is when she realized that this is not only a physical battle with an invisible virus. It is higher than what we can understand in medicine; it is a spiritual battle against God's crown of creation: humanity. It was absolutely an evil plan by using God's given intelligence with wrong motives to create diseases to multiply death, disguised as "scientific research" and letting people die without early intervention. What a crime. What a tragedy.

Thoughts rushed through the billions of neurons in my brain that day. The Frontline Doctors' voices stirred up my emotions as I reflected on the persecution I suffered. Simply because I used my critical thinking, knowledge, and experience gained from thirty-plus years of providing patient care. It deeply troubled me to think that those in authority set restrictions on me for doing my job. For doing everything possible to help people suffering from Covid and making them feel better. For using my judgment in making clinical decisions to save lives from a deadly virus. A virus that we now know was studied in a research lab in Wuhan—one with the potency to kill millions around the world. The full scope of this tragedy has yet to unfold.

The Greatest Failure

Earlier, I mentioned my chance meeting with Dr. Robert Malone. In a recent Substack post he wrote that "virtually all who read our essays and books, or listen to my many podcasts, are aware of the profound failures, medical mismanagement, notable ethical breaches, and deep corruption that characterize the medical system and public health response to the COVID crisis. We are also aware that the various branches of the US medical system, pharmaceutical-industrial complex and the US Government/HHS system has deployed a wide range of propaganda, censorship, and PsyWar tools and technologies to both block citizens and medical care providers from communicating about these failures and from proposing alternative solutions."[22]

He went on to discuss how an independent survey of the US healthcare system by the New York-based Commonwealth Fund for 2021–23 showed that the system is failing citizens of the United States. Malone insists that federal interference in the healthcare market had failed to achieve any of its objectives, with the US ranking last among ten countries in regard to access to care, processes, administrative efficiencies, equity, and health outcomes. What's worse, Malone says the survey shows that US residents are paying the most money for the worst overall outcomes.[23]

This failure to heal brings to mind the Bible verse where Martha expressed regret over her brother (Lazarus) dying because no help was available to alleviate his suffering: "Now Martha said to Jesus, 'Lord, if You had been here, my brother would not have died'" (John 11:21). Like Martha in Lazarus's powerful story, I harbored apprehension and great regret in my heart. If more of my colleagues in primary care had been practicing healing medicine, with great compassion for their suffering patients, millions would not have died across the world because of lack of treatment.

We clearly saw the dark defects in many souls during the early days of the pandemic. People panicked over not being able to find a doctor to prescribe early treatment. Those who did often had to run from pharmacy to pharmacy in their weakened condition in hopes of getting a prescription filled. We saw the moral deficiencies and

---

22 Robert W. Malone, MD, "US Healthcare during COVID- Lowest Performance, Highest Cost: The best of times for 'the system,' the worst of times for patients," September 19, 2024, https://www.malone.news/p/us-healthcare-during-covid-lowest.

23 Ibid.

malignancies when patients were refused treatment; pharmacies refused to fill prescriptions at the time when victims needed them the most because their lungs were deteriorating rapidly. Unethical approaches became the "standard of care" during the pandemic.

In his major book-length expose, The Wuhan Cover-Up, one-time presidential candidate (and New York Times bestselling author) Robert F. Kennedy Jr. nailed down the fact that we faced cruelty from something much bigger than we at first thought: "Whatever the reason, bioweapons science has been a moral wasteland since its inception, and modern gain-of-function and vaccine research are irrevocably hobbled to the bioweapons-industrial complex." [24]

The emphasis on fighting the coronavirus did not fall on early diagnosis and treatment. Health authorities did not conduct a massive educational program for the public and medical practitioners to teach them about the disease process and early diagnoses of Covid. They did not disseminate knowledge so people could learn how treatment worked if initiated in the first five to seven days. There were no community-based clinics providing early treatment for the public. No education for primary care providers about the outpatient treatment protocols for symptomatic infections. No education on health promotion and disease prevention for high-risk health workers, high-risk teachers, and nursing home patients.

Instead, we observed intense, dictatorial methods employed at the local, state, and federal level. Immediate, widespread lockdowns of hospitals, public schools, libraries, businesses, places of worship, and countless other facilities revolutionized daily life overnight. Yet, with early treatment there would not have been any reason to shutter nearly every public place affecting our lives (ironically, although millions couldn't go to church, they could visit their neighborhood liquor store).

---

[24] Robert F. Kennedy Jr., *The Wuhan Cover-Up and the Terrifying Bioweapons Arms Race* (Children's Health Defense, Skyhorse, December 5, 2023), 88.

On top of all this needless activity, professional care providers were persecuted for demonstrating compassion for the suffering, saving lives, educating the public, and speaking the truth. I will never forget the tyranny and cruelty behind such actions. Indeed, there were no reasons for health authorities to revoke my license, which I studied hard for many years to obtain. Then I used that license to help society's most vulnerable members, often at my own expense. Nor was I compensated for the late-night services I offered to virus victims, many lacking any other kind of medical treatment.

Because I prescribed medicines for off-label use (which I had done for more than two decades for similar symptoms), I lost my license. Still, I understood—as many other doctors did—that we were fighting a spiritual war with physical manifestations. Jesus said in John: "The thief does not come except to steal, and to kill, and to destroy. I have come that they may have life, and that they may have it more abundantly" (John 10:10). In my case, the thief had come, but the Lord would restore what he tried to steal.

Chapter 6

Touching a Nerve

In chapter 5 I talked about the divine appointments that led me to various quarters of the world in less than a year. When my travels began with the visit to the US Supreme Court—with prominent doctors, experts, and scientists fighting for freedom in medicine in our nation—I couldn't hold back the tears. Hearing their voices speaking up for the truth and feeling their emotional pain expressing the urgent need to awaken this great nation touched a nerve deep within.

Pictures of the agony of living under communism in my native Romania immediately sprang to mind. So did thoughts of the oppression, persecution, humiliation, character assassination, intimidation, tyranny, and propaganda. Unless you have lived under a communist regime, it's hard to grasp the indignities of never being able to freely express one's values and beliefs. Growing up, the fear of communist cruelty always gripped my heart. I knew they regularly threw people in prison for sharing their faith and standing up for the truth. I lived with the uncertainty throughout my younger years and adolescence. Now, three decades later, I was standing in my adopted nation's capital as a voice, speaking out against the same persecution I had seen in my youth.

I sacrificed everything to be able to escape from communists and live in this great and free nation. But facing the health care system's hardball tactics left me feeling the same kind of humiliation, intimidation, and oppression. Persecuted again in what is supposed to a free country, and all because I used my critical thinking to make clinical decisions. When I decided to go to nursing school after arriving in the US, I hungered to learn how to provide holistic care to suffering people. Thirsting for more knowledge, I admired the professors, scientists, instructors, and mentors who shared their knowledge, experience, and expertise.

Like a sponge, my brain absorbed all the information to the maximum. I looked forward to putting into practice everything that I learned on a daily basis. I intended to treat patients with the same kind of love and dedication that my teachers and mentors had given to me. I loved true science. I read thousands of articles written by top experts in medicine and published in the most prestigious medical journals. I also devoured magazines and books written by professional health care providers.

In addition, I participated in hundreds of medical conferences and got thousands of hours of continuing medical education in more than thirty years of practice as a nurse, nurse practitioner, and then as a doctor of nursing practice. Over time, I became an expert in health care myself. Medicine and patient care became part of my DNA. I felt that my mission on this earth was to help patients feel better and save their lives whenever possible.

Caring for the Suffering

Caring for suffering patients in multiple roles over thirty-plus years, I felt that I gave a piece of my heart to each one of them. For eight years during the 1990s we had suffering patients living in our home. I spent day and night with them, meeting physical and psychological needs. I went as far as providing care in great details, even small interventions, such as placing some vitamin A & D ointment on dry lips or a few drops of water to release discomfort of patients suffering from a high fever.

I also provided end-of-life care, spending time at the bedsides of dying people. I often held a dying person's hand so they did not have to die alone. I prayed with them when there was no pastor, priest, or loved ones nearby when their soul departed from this earth. It is impossible to come out of such experiences with dry eyes. Given this history, I was astonished during the onset of the pandemic that health authorities told physicians to avoid early interventions and let patients suffer because "there is no treatment for Covid." Every life is precious.

My education and experience in the health care system led me to gain more knowledge and understanding about life on earth. Here is a short description of my background. Back in Romania I completed a college education in 1986 and earned my Bachelor of Economic Sciences degree at The Academy of Economic Sciences in Bucharest. After arriving in the US in 1990, I first assimilated into American life by improving my proficiency in English and then setting out to complete extensive medical studies.

I earned a Bachelor of Science in Nursing in 1999 from the Oregon Health & Science University (OHSU), a public research university in Portland whose main campus includes two hospitals (founded in 1887 as the University of Oregon Medical Department, it later became the University of Oregon Medical School). Following that, I completed a master's degree program with training in internal medicine at Kaiser Permanente in Clackamas. Later I received clinical training at OHSU's endocrinology division, did cardiology consulting at St. Vincent's Medical Center, and did primary care at the Veterans Affairs Medical Center in Portland. Finally, at OHSU I earned my Doctor of Nursing Practice, a PhD-level degree with clinical orientation and a focus on metabolic syndrome (hypertension, diabetes, dyslipidemia) in primary care practice.

As an ANP (Adult Nurse Practitioner) and GNP (Geriatric Nurse Practitioner) with prescriptive authority and DEA licensing—meaning I could prescribe controlled substances—I practiced general medicine for more than twenty years. As mentioned earlier, I provided care to minorities, the homeless, and other marginalized or needy people. I volunteered more than fifteen thousand hours at two community health clinics in Portland. During the pandemic, I treated hundreds of patients suffering from Covid, saving their lives with early interventions using safe, well-known medications.

I am also the founder and former CEO/operator of two memory care facilities, where I provided physical, emotional, and spiritual care (including comfort care at the end of life) to patients with multiple chronic conditions. I am a board member of Star of Hope USA, which supports children with disabilities and their families—financially, emotionally, and spiritually. I have also written three books: *Find Your Peace* (Charisma House, 2019); *Created In His Image with Unique Purpose* (Trilogy Christian Publishing, 2021) and *Covid-19, Post Covid-19, Alleviate the Fear* (Trilogy Christian Publishing, 2021). (All are available at www.rodicamalos.com).

Lacking Guidelines

Despite having the best professors, educators, and mentors in Oregon's leading academic setting, during pandemic time we lacked guidelines and protocols in primary care for patients with Covid symptoms. So, I relied on my knowledge from those long years of education, health care experience, and expertise in working with patients with acute and multiple chronic conditions. I also learned from the most knowledgeable experts, including top doctors in the US and the world, who had compassion for the suffering and developed protocols to treat them early and save their lives.

As Brian Tyson, George Fareed, and Matthew Crawford stated in the previously-mentioned book, *Overcoming the COVID Darkness:* "By following our effective protocol (patients) were also able to witness extraordinary improvements and the resolution of symptoms in our patients. The gratitude and testimonials we have received have been prolific, and we know in our hearts that there is no reason for doctors to modify successful and life-saving treatments just to pacify the naysayers, pessimists, and unbelievers brainwashed by national agencies.

"Sadly, some medical academics published patently false information early on, which you will learn more about in this book. Many flawed clinical trials were guided and published by individuals with vast conflicts of interest. Unfortunately, their ulterior motives were never disclosed. To appease these fraudulent academics, medical institutions and official agencies essentially blocked all early treatment protocols. Meanwhile, we couldn't bear to witness the dire consequences of withholding treatment—not as we saw other patients go into respiratory failure and die on ventilators alone, without the basic human right of having their loved ones by their side."[25]

Later, Dr. Tyson added: "It's unconscionable that early treatment was not being offered for something that was actually a 'super' virus: genetically enhanced in a laboratory and made much more likely to be extraordinarily dangerous for humans. ... Despite the success of the HCQ treatment protocol, and despite the 100 (percent) success rate for our patients who were treated early, the unthinkable happened: the NIH, FDA, WHO, and CDC knowingly blocked effective early treatment for a virus enhanced in a lab to infect and kill humans."[26]

Reinforcing Mandates

Looking back, the words I would describe about government vaccine mandates are terms like "harsh," "oppressive," and "unethical." Health care workers in the health field, caring for patients face-to-face, were forced to get vaccinated against coronavirus. The majority of us did so because we had always believed in obeying the law. As always, we trusted the authorities, the education system, and scientists with all our heart.

Given this background, it never crossed our minds that something would go wrong with all the measures the state implemented for everyone's safety. But when the first group of hundreds of health care providers from hospitals and clinics lined up outside the building in a huge parking lot area, we faced strict security

---

[25] *Overcoming the COVID Darkness*, 22–24.

[26] Ibid., 36-37

measures. They checked our picture IDs to get the antivirus shot, with the staff distributing envelopes containing papers of background information about the vaccine. When we arrived at the door to enter in the building, other personnel collected those envelopes. We did not have adequate time to read (ten to twenty or more pages) while in line. As I contemplated what was going on, anxiety, uncertainty, and fearful thoughts rushed through my mind. I knew that the vaccines had not been fully studied through all the necessary phases and scientifically proven as "safe and effective."

When the woman at the entrance asked me to give her back the envelope so she could toss it into a huge garbage bin, my instincts told me that something was not normal. It felt so sinister. In medicine, when it comes to consenting to a procedure or treatment, we like to review information completely in order to make a well-informed decision. Not this time. Fear gripped my heart because we were being forced to get a vaccine injected into our body without knowing anything about potential side effects. Without studies completed to insure the best scientific procedures would be carried out. Without completed research. This kind of unscientific approach was unacceptable to most people in the medical field.

For more than thirty years in medicine, I had learned to always educate patients about safety procedures, interventions, side effects, and potential adverse effects of medication that would enter their body. Now we were handed papers in line and moments later asked to give them back. We barely had time to open the envelope with a stack of pages, let alone read them to understand the medication we would receive through an invasive procedure that delivered chemicals to our muscles. What changed that now? We were herded like "sheep to the slaughter," unable to say anything. Like robots going through the motions, we went through the door and past computers carrying only our ID in our hands. The strict security in place gave it a very strange atmosphere. Still, the health care system mandated that all medical professionals submit to such treatment. It shook my faith in the academic and health care system I had trusted in for so long.

Ignoring Standard Practice

Ironically, we who were hands-on in providing direct patient care received dictates from authorities who provided no care to those suffering from COVID-19. In the past, if patients had respiratory problems, viruses, bacteria, allergies, asthma, pneumonia, or COPD, we gave them oral agents. Then, if necessary, bronchodilators and corticosteroids via nebulizers to help reduce inflammation in their lungs, and oxygen to help them breathe and aid their recovery.

If they had a high fever we gave them anti-fever medications. If they had inflammation in connective tissue when their immune system overreacted, we gave them immunomodulators, which are medicines that change the immune system to help it work more effectively. If they had a viral infection we gave them anti-viral meds to reduce the viral load. If they had bacterial infections, we gave them antibiotics. If they were at risk of developing blood clots, we gave them prophylactic anticoagulants.

Given these procedures, I asked myself and other physicians why we could not use the same approach during pandemic time, when death was knocking at every door. Instead, high-ranking health authorities told us to give no treatment, no prophylactics, no training, and no education. The only news we heard repeatedly concerned the numbers of how many people were infected and how many had died.

During this sinister time, I often reflected about how in the past we had provided direct care to our patients. We attended to so many details with their physical needs, taking them to the bathroom, changing diapers every two hours if necessary, and transferring them to a wheelchair for mobility three or four times a day. We cared for their personal hygiene, manually fed them if needed, and helped them with all activities of daily living. And now if a deathly-ill patient asked for help, I was to say: "Sorry, there is no treatment for Covid"?

Such stark realities and such obvious contrasts to normal medical procedures stabbed at me with the symbolic force of a dozen steak knives. I became restless in my soul and spirit, even losing sleep over those lies and dictatorial methods. They brought to mind the communists who didn't care for peoples' lives. In my mind, the parallels to communism were so apparent it caused me great disturbance and discomfort. Something inside of me was telling me that it was completely unacceptable to let people die from a disease that could be prevented with early treatment. It bothered me greatly to wonder: How many lives could have been saved with early treatment? How many people would be alive today if safe medications had been repurposed and used as off-label treatments, instead of being banned by authorities during the onset of the pandemic?

The same questions should trouble everyone reading this book.

Chapter 7

Not a Single Word

As you know by now, I abhorred the variety of medically unsound approaches recommended by health care authorities during the pandemic. The one that caused me the most trouble was spreading the idea that there was no treatment for Covid. If that weren't bad enough, sending people to the ER only when their symptoms had worsened to the point they couldn't breathe was a practice I considered unconscionable.

As bad as all that was, when I received the nursing board's letter of license revocation, I felt as if my world was collapsing. I knew I had done the best I could to help suffering patients feel better during their times of desperation. Indeed, I had done nothing wrong. What was I to do when I heard the agony in every patient's voice, alone and isolated and crying for help during my telemedicine conferences? I went the extra mile and even sacrificed personal time and expense to help them overcome this monstrous virus that killed millions. What's worse was the propaganda that spread around the world, instilling fear in people's minds and hearts and making them think another pandemic was imminent. Making them think they had been sentenced to die.

At the small clinic where I worked, our mission statement said that we provided care with the love of Jesus Christ. That was my mission too. I could not ignore the cry of patients in our community who were in such terrible distress. In my brain and heart, I deeply sensed their emotional pain. As I put myself in their shoes, I could sense their psychological pain too. I regularly asked myself, "What would Jesus do when a sick patient asked for help?" Often in reply the

Lord's words from Matthew 25:40 would echo through my mind: "Inasmuch as you did it to one of the least of these My brethren, you did it to Me."

To further my level of care, I constantly checked medical resources for more information in order to educate myself about available treatments. I took one hundred continuing education hours (required for license renewal) from the top experts in the academic world. I looked specifically for treatments for patients suffering from Covid and found none. Those infected with coronavirus were the most vulnerable at risk to die if not treated early, in the first three to five days. This was especially true of victims with other comorbidities, which is the presence of two or more health conditions, such as kidney disease and diabetes, or heart disease and asthma.

We had relatives and friends who had already died from Covid, along with some well-known members of the community. The question that persistently ran through my mind: "How long should I wait for solutions?" Day and night I thought about the mess we were in and the threat to my nurse practitioner's license if I started to treat suffering patients. What a paradox! Throughout my time in medical studies and during my practical experience, I learned how to make patients feel better. To think that we were to "do nothing" went against the grain of every class I took, every mentor who counseled me, and every practice rooted in the Hippocratic Oath. To stand still and watch people die needlessly was the worst nightmare of my entire professional career.

Every day was a challenge. I could not stand to see suffering patients not getting the help they needed, with the medications that could help them feel better and save their lives, comforting their entire family. It may sound basic, but it wasn't until after I treated the first patient that I gained a profound awareness of how treating the patient was providing treatment for the whole family. Helping the entire family was my goal. Earlier I mentioned the verse from Matthew 25:40: "Inasmuch as you did it to one of the least of these My brethren, you did it to Me." Another verse from the same book also resounded in my mind: "And whoever gives one of these little ones only a cup of cold water in the name of a disciple, assuredly, I say to you, he shall by no means lose his reward" (Matt. 10:42)

Irrational Restrictions

One day I thought about the restrictions placed on us that prohibited us from visiting the sick. The restriction collided with Christ's admonition to those lacking compassion: "I was a stranger and you did not take Me in, naked and you did not clothe Me, sick and in prison and you did not visit Me" (Matt. 25:43). Where did the idea that we were not to visit the sick or suffering originate?

When the nursing board investigated me, one of their accusations was that I visited a family of frail people in their late eighties. The husband and wife were both wasting away in isolation from Covid. They were getting progressively weaker and lethargic. Their cognitive skills and ability to concentrate were also in decline, leaving them with what we called "foggy brain."

The woman's blood oxygen level had dropped to 91 percent (normal is 98 to 100), but she didn't even realize her blood oxygen was so low. She was more concerned that her husband get to the hospital. Despite his neurological deficit, poor cognition, dizziness, and poor body balance, after going to the ER he had been sent back home with little treatment.

I noticed little food or other supplies in their home, but then they were too weak to cook. They thought they did not need to eat much because their taste and smell had been so severely affected by the virus, leaving them with little appetite. They told friends and family "we have everything we need" so nobody would worry about them. When I arrived at their house, I discovered a radically different story. Elderly people were the most neglected during the early stages of the pandemic. Isolation represented a huge handicap for them. It increased their emotional pain and psychological distress, leading many down the path of decline and death.

At that visit, I had a nebulizer with me in my bag. A nebulizer is a small machine that converts liquid medication into a mist, allowing patients to inhale it through a mouthpiece or a mask. It is often used to treat people with lung diseases, such as asthma, chronic obstructive pulmonary disease (COPD), or chronic lung disease. I knew from experience that a nebulizer is the most helpful method to reduce inflammation in the lungs for anyone suffering from respiratory distress or breathing difficulties, like this elderly couple. This would allow these patients to breathe better, improve their oxygen levels, and prevent Covid pneumonia.

I showed them how to use the nebulizer with budesonide solution; as I watched, the woman's blood oxygen level went from 91 percent to 97 percent. The improvement allowed us to enjoy a pleasant conversation. On that visit, I also dropped off some homecooked food for this couple. This increased their energy levels, greatly improved their morale, and literally saved their lives.

Questioning My Visits

The investigator asked me a few times why I visited sick people at home and if my boss knew about my visits. That question disturbed me deep inside. I responded by asking her what happened to the idea of "loving our neighbor" by caring for them and helping them, especially during their serious sickness at such an unsettled time in our nation's history. My boss, Dr. Sayson, was also a strong believer and visited vulnerable patients when they were too weak to leave their home on a regular basis. He helped the sick to get better and prayed for every one of them. This brought incredible solace to the suffering patients and the entire family in the comfort of their own home.

Quite frankly, I did not understand the investigator's question. I was shocked when she questioned my visits to these vulnerable people at my own expense. Not only did I not charge them, I didn't invoice any health insurers or Medicare for such treatments. After all, are we supposed to allow old people to die in isolation? A friend from another church we had once attended told me of an elderly man from that church who was found dead in his home after isolating himself, but had no neighbors or health care professionals stopping by to check on his wellbeing.

Not only was that heartbreaking news, the investigator's voice resounded in my mind: "Why did you visit the patients at home?" It left me wondering, "Why? Why? Why?" Even as I write these words my eyes are filled with tears. My entire life I had compassion for the sick. From a young age, I had learned from Scripture that we are to visit the sick and help others.

Now, spiritually I understood exactly what was going on. At this time, demonic forces were attacking humanity. I did not know that I was not supposed to visit patients whom I had known for more than three decades, ever since my days as a university student in Bucharest. I knew many sick families from the Romanian immigrant community, from elderly grandparents down to their toddler grandchildren. Someone asking me why I visited those who were sick and needed my help the most made me want to protest: "Why would I not visit them?" I will never forget the atrocities that were committed against the powerless and weak old people during the pandemic. It reminded me of the suffering many had to endure under communism and made me wonder if they were the victims of indirect persecution.

Another question from the investigator shocked me too: "Why didn't you ask about their vaccination status?" What difference would that make to a patient sick with compromised lungs, who could can only speak in halting phrases because of shortness of breath? Who was tired by every breath they took and was unable to concentrate? Who was I to discriminate between vaccinated and unvaccinated patients? I thought of the irony of getting vaccinated per the health care system's mandate and when I contracted Covid, my doctor did not treat me anyway. I had to find a private doctor via telemedicine. Fortunately, this doctor had compassion for the sick and prescribed medication for me and my husband that helped us feel better and prevented our hospitalization and premature death.

Seeking Treatment

I explained to the investigator that asking an old Romanian person about being vaccinated for Covid was culturally insensitive when people knew that the vaccine was experimental. And, that people were misinformed or disinformed about side effects and knew the vaccines had not been studied for a long time regarding possible complications. People from different cultures were skeptical of vaccines under such circumstances.

I learned in school that we needed to be aware of a patient's vaccination status. But what if these patients were sick with Covid, needed treatment right away, and did not have the energy to talk at length and give me a medical history? A deadly virus had taken their energy away, caused neurological deficits, and made them so lethargic they were unable to get up from bed and even go to the bathroom. Those were acute conditions that needed immediate treatment to prevent further complications. A vaccine given when people are sick can worsen their condition and can sometimes be lethal.

Many physician friends were told to give "nothing" in their setting for people sentenced to die from this lethal virus. Dictatorship was alive and well in the medical field in those days, dictating that doctors not treat suffering patients—the most vulnerable people during the pandemic. I can testify that not since my days under communism had I ever witnessed such a terrible battle against the truth. The fear of communism gripped my heart all over again.

Spirit of Fear

During pandemic time, the term COVID-19 hurtled across the world in an instant. Whether it was local, national, or international news, pandemic awareness spread across TV, the internet, social media, newspapers, and radio. We heard about it everywhere we went, whether in the grocery store, at work, or in conversation with coworkers, friends, relatives, or family. The result: instilling fear in people's minds and spirits, leaving millions feeling overwhelmed and stressed out. Fear is the greatest enemy of our health, both physically and spiritually.

Emotions of fear will stir up negative thoughts. In turn, this toll will lead to anxiety and sadness, causing a shift in neurotransmitters and neurochemicals released in our body. Levels of such mood elevators as serotonin, dopamine, melatonin, and other neuro-chemicals decrease and lead to depression. That can cause lack of sleep, leading to sleep deprivation, which weakens the immune system.

Throughout my life, I have learned faith is the antidote to fear, but Dr. David Levy, whom I mentioned in my talk at the Romanian Parliament in chapter 4, does a particularly good job detailing this in his video, "Fear in Crisis."[27] He discusses how fear affects people's brains, the immune system, and the entire body during the pandemic. He explains how fear also triggers thoughts and emotions that send signals to the brain that danger is coming. It sends messages to the pituitary gland, which starts the process of secreting adrenocortico-tropic hormones, stimulating the adrenal gland to release cortisol and epinephrine.

When fear increases, the heart rate increases. The most dangerous effect of this is the cortisol that suppresses the immune system. The immune system helps the body to fight against bacteria, microorganisms, and viruses. Fearful thoughts and the emotions created by fear increased the chances of getting the virus by lowering the immune system that fights viral infections, including COVID-19. The thoughts of fear are like poison for the mind and the body, occupying our mind and taking up "real estate" in our brain, which has billions of neurons.

When we continue to repeat those thoughts of fear in our mind throughout the day, fear will control our mind. This weakens the

---

[27] Dr. David Levy, *"Fear in Crisis* – Part 1 (Coronavirus COVID-19) Help for Anxiety," YouTube, https://www.youtube.com/watch?v=nfrbm1dvZaI, accessed November 20, 2020.

immune system and leaves it ineffective against fighting the virus or bacteria, which causes more damage to our body, soul, and spirit. Spiritually, we know who wants to destroy our life with thoughts of fear and uncertainty. Although I mentioned this verse at the end of chapter 5, it merits repeating here: "The thief does not come except to steal, and to kill, and to destroy. I have come that they may have life, and that they may have it more abundantly" (John 10:10). Whenever we are fighting a battle with fear, we can be sure the enemy of our souls is behind it.

I have come to the understanding that the battle with thoughts of fear and despair is very real, a palpable enemy that can make the hairs on your neck stand up. Fear and panic, stirred by the "invisible enemy" for several years now, led to increased levels of stress. In turn, that caused an increase in cortisol (the stress hormone) and other neurotransmitters, affecting our mind and the ability to think and make decisions. All body systems were affected by an unhealthy amount of neurochemicals released in the body during these stressful years.

All systems connected to our brain are affected by increased levels of stress from fear, causing depression with all its consequences. During the pandemic, all of the people I talked to—but especially patients with COVID-19—expressed fear, worry, and anxiety. Many reported thoughts of depression when we interacted on a regular basis during their sickness. This all started on January 22, 2020, when the first case of COVID-19 (a novel coronavirus named SARS-CoV-2 that originated in Wuhan, China in December 2019) was reported in the US, and followed for years afterward.

Moved with Compassion

Given the deprivation we suffered in my childhood, my heart has always moved with compassion for those who suffered physically and psychologically from different illnesses. This was especially for those stricken by the deadly virus and post-COVID-19 symptoms. Like many medical providers, when the discussion about coronavirus started in the US in early 2020, I believed this was "just "another virus." One we could control with our advanced knowledge in science, experience in medicine, and pharmaceutical technology. At the time, I didn't doubt that the virus would be controlled (with the top expertise in health), nor did I realize that it would be that aggressive and unpredictable, killing millions globally. And I did not know that health care professionals would feel so helpless and hopeless.

As the news of people dying by the thousands in a short time catapulted around the world, fear mounted in people's minds and hearts. Alarming daily news reports became a plague in themself, making people panic from fear of COVID-19. But those who fear the Lord run to Him in such a time like this to find refuge and safety. They know that:

- "The name of the LORD is a fortified tower; the righteous run to it and are safe" (Prov. 18:10 NIV).
- God is love and in Him there is no fear: "For God gave us a spirit not of fear but of power and love and self-control" (2 Tim. 1:7 ESV).
- God is always with us. "Fear not, for I am with you; be not dismayed, for I am your God. I will strengthen you, yes, I will help you, I will uphold you with My righteous right hand" (Isa. 41:10).

While anxiety and depression from COVID-19 put a mark on people's lives, God's prescription is always stronger. His powerful Word offers us reassurance. The fear of dying cripples people; increased anxiety and depression were observed since the start of COVID-19.

Anxiety, depression, and other neurocognitive disorders were not strange to me because of more than three decades of experience in memory care facilities. I provided prolonged hours of care to residents with different kinds of dementia and increased anxiety and depression.

Fear, anxiety, and depression increased when people were advised in the beginning that if they got COVID-19 symptoms, they needed to stay home and if their symptoms grew worse, to call their primary care provider to let them know about the symptoms so they could be screened by telephone for the virus. And/or to call 911 to get hospitalized for treatment, creating the "hospital-dependent for COVID-19" model. It sounded like a strange model to me, knowing that for thirty-plus years we had provided care to people in a homelike environment in a community-based care setting to keep people out of the hospital.

But as I learned, when it came to COVID-19, there was nothing sane about the health care system's approach.

Chapter 8

A Gap in Primary Care

During the pandemic, there were no early treatment protocols in primary care for patients suffering from the lethal pathogen. Living in the most advanced nation in the world, the very thought sickened me. It even struck me as sinister. My heart broke for patients isolated at home and cowering in fear because primary care providers were so limited in the tools available to us. While there were over-the-counter (OTC) medications, herbal preparations, and home remedies available, none were appropriate to fight this deadly virus.

Because so many people were waiting too long to get interventions in time, some started to develop pneumonia (see the letter in chapter 3 from the family pastors with their heartbreaking testimony). In many cases, when the patients had other comorbidities, it was difficult to treat empirically at home. Their fears increased with the worsening of every symptom. Medical providers in hospitals learned from their own experience to treat acute symptoms based on the pathophysiology caused by the COVID-19 virus. Only in a primary care setting were we encouraged to tell patients to care for themselves at home. They were to use OTC preparations and home remedies until their symptoms got worse, and then to go to the hospital. Repeating this makes me shake my head. Telling people to follow this kind of regimen brings to mind tales of nineteenth century snake charmers in a Wild West traveling medicine show.

As primary care providers, we could have learned from hospital interventions that could have been adapted for use at home to prevent hospitalization and death. At this point I despaired for those suffering with multiple COVID-19 symptoms. I could give them nothing but God's promises:

- "Fear not, for I have redeemed you; I have called you by your name; you are Mine. When you pass through the waters, I will be with you; and through the rivers, they shall not overflow you. When you walk through the fire, you shall not be burned, nor shall the flame scorch you" (Isa. 43:1–2).
- "Be strong and of good courage, do not fear nor be afraid of them; for the LORD your God, He is the One who goes with you. He will not leave you nor forsake you. ... And the LORD, He is the One who goes before you. He will be with you, He will not leave you nor forsake you; do not fear nor be dismayed" (Deut. 31: 6 and 8).
- God's direction to Paul: "And He said to me, 'My grace is sufficient for you, for My strength is made perfect in weakness.' Therefore most gladly I will rather boast in my infirmities, that the power of Christ may rest upon me" (2 Cor. 12:9).

Trusting in God

I offered these Scriptures not as some kind of magic medicine, but in recognition of the vital importance of trusting in God for our physical and spiritual health. We should rejoice in the fact that He is our help in time of need. He is our Protector, holding us with His mighty hand and giving us strength in terrible times, be that a pandemic, a hurricane, or a wildfire. God's promises are like seeds, with power for exponential multiplication to increase our faith in Him and our hope for getting through difficult issues.

Sadness and depression only deepen the sickness in our body, affecting all systems down to the bones. In effect they deplete our body of energy and strength. As Proverbs says: "A cheerful heart is good medicine, but a crushed spirit dries up the bones" (Prov. 17:22 NIV). The dreary days of lockdowns and restrictions that stayed in place for a year—or even two years in some areas after the worst had lessened—crushed our national spirit. This left our citizens with dried up bones and no solutions in sight, except for God's mercy.

The "sicken-in-place" paradigm came about because of a lack of randomized, controlled clinical studies and scientific information. In turn, that led to a lack of guidance and protocols for early intervention in primary care settings. This dreadful situation left general practitioners in primary care practices without solutions to treat COVID-19 patients and alleviate their fears. We so desperately wanted to prevent our patients from suffering panic attacks that would affect far more, including their immunity and health conditions. We knew these could lead to even more frightening symptoms and an increased fear of death.

As the weeks went by and the gloom of lockdowns settled over the nation, I started to receive calls from very sick people in our community. They were so exhausted from COVID-19 symptoms they could barely speak. Yet, I could still hear the panic in their voices, especially those who were afraid to call their provider because they were so sick and terrified of going to the hospital and getting placed on a ventilator, only to die in isolation.

Many patients reported that they had heard on the news and social media of that very thing happening because hospitals were filled with patients suffering from COVID-19. I could hear the agony in their voices when they called, begging for treatment for their symptoms.

Looking for Answers

Determined to help patients suffering from terrible symptoms, I started to search for any study that would address early interventions at home. I wanted to find potential solutions for the hurting. One of the first came from a medical journal with a good reputation: The American Journal of Medicine. An article that first appeared online in August of 2020 recognized that approximately nine months of coronavirus-2 spreading worldwide had led to widespread acute hospitalizations and death.

"The rapidity and highly communicable nature of the SARS-CoV-2 outbreak has hampered the design and execution of definitive randomized controlled trials of therapy outside of the clinic or hospital," wrote Dr. Peter McCullough, who headed a team of 21 physicians who worked on the study.

"The rapidity and highly communicable nature of the SARS-CoV-2 outbreak has hampered the design and execution of definitive randomized, controlled trials of therapy outside of the clinic or hospital. In the absence of clinical trial results, physicians must use what has been learned about the pathophysiology of SARS-CoV-2 infection in determining early outpatient treatment of the illness with the aim of preventing hospitalization or death.

"This article outlines key pathophysiological principles that relate to the patient with early infection treated at home. Therapeutic approaches based on these principles include 1) reduction of reinoculation, 2) combination antiviral therapy, 3) immune-modulation, 4) antiplatelet/antithrombotic therapy, and 5) administration of oxygen, monitoring, and telemedicine."[28]

At last! I had found reputable physicians who were saying early treatment at home was possible! Previously, I had faced the same alarming and scary situation as every general practitioner in primary care—the inability to save lives through early intervention. Professional people in hospitals learned quickly about the disease caused by the COVID-19 infection's pathophysiology, as they were exposed to so many severe cases and had developed protocols. These protocols were based on information gathered throughout this time about the advanced pathophysiology caused by the virus in hospital settings.

---

[28] Peter A. McCullough, MD, et. al., "Pathophysiological Basis and Rationale for Early Outpatient Treatment of SARS-CoV-2 (COVID-19) Infection," The American Journal of Medicine, Vol. 134, Issue 1, January 2021, 16-22, printed online at Science Direct, https://www.sciencedirect.com/science/article/pii/ S0002934320306732.

Still, some people continued to die because they got to the hospital too late, after their symptoms had worsened. This had caused further damage to the lungs and other organs, already under attack from the inflammatory process caused by the virus. It started to aggressively multiply in the lungs and the entire body while the patient was waiting at home due to "sicken-in-place" recommendations. How sad, since this could have been prevented.

An Intense Battle

Suddenly I found myself immersed in an intense battle to prevent further disaster in our community. The struggle throughout the entire world was evident: the uncertainty and frustrations regarding the true origins of the virus and the mechanism of spreading it throughout the entire world. And, the lack of expertise in knowing the infection's pathophysiology. This was something we needed to know in order to treat the disease caused by this aggressive virus, particularly among a segment of the population with other underlying conditions.

Just one month into the new year of 2020—on January 31—the US government banned outside entry into the country and issued a proclamation to prevent risk of further transmission of the virus and to prevent further disaster in the USA. Years later, re-reading just a small portion of the announcement sends chills up my spine:

"Coronaviruses are a large family of viruses. Some cause illness in people and others circulate among animals, including camels, cats, and bats. Animal coronaviruses are capable of evolving to infect people and subsequently spreading through human-to-human transmission. This occurred with both Middle East Respiratory Syndrome and SARS. Many of the individuals with the earliest confirmed cases of 2019-nCoV in Wuhan, China had some link to a large seafood and live animal market, suggesting animal-to-human transmission. Later, a growing number of infected individuals reportedly did not have exposure to animal markets, indicating human-to-human transmission. Chinese officials now report that sustained human-to-human transmission of the virus is occurring in China. Manifestations of severe disease have included severe pneumonia, acute respiratory distress syndrome, septic shock, and multi-organ failure."[29]

Top leaders in our nation criticized President Donald Trump for being too prudent in his action to keep Americans safe from a vicious virus that could kill millions. In addition, the news media created tension with widespread reporting of these criticisms, leading to more struggles among citizens who now feared the pandemic in even greater proportions. In his book on the pandemic's affects on the 2020 election, publisher and author Stephen Strang noted that "according to The Hill, on January 31, 2020, Speaker of the House Nancy Pelosi said President Trump's decision to extend the travel ban to six African nations was 'outrageous, unAmerican and threatened the rule of law.' That statement didn't age well. In addition, the World Health Organization (WHO) tweeted on January 14 that there was no clear evidence of human-to-human transmission of the virus, but by January 23 the organization said human-to-human transmission was occurring."[30]

Several weeks after that head-spinning turnaround by the WHO, the same organization declared the novel coronavirus (COVID-19) outbreak a global pandemic: "At a news briefing, WHO Director-General, Dr. Tedros Adhanom Ghebreyesus, noted that over the past (two) weeks, the number of cases outside China increased (thirteen-fold) and the number of countries with cases increased threefold. Further increases are expected. He said that the WHO is 'deeply concerned both by the alarming levels of spread and severity and by the alarming levels of inaction,' and he called on countries to take

---

[29] "Proclamation on Suspension of Entry as Immigrants and Nonimmigrants of Persons who Pose a Risk of Transmitting 2019 Novel Coronavirus," White House healthcare directive, January 31, 2020, https://trumpwhitehouse.archives.gov/presidential-actions/proclamation-suspension-entry-immigrants-nonimmigrants-persons-pose-risk-transmitting-2019-novel-coronavirus/

[30] Stephen E. Strang, *God, Trump, and COVID-19*: How the Pandemic is Affecting Christians, the World, and America's 2020 Election (Charisma House, 2020,) xi.

action now to contain the virus. 'We should double down,' he said. 'We should be more aggressive.'"[31]

The Battle Continues

The battle with uncertainty and unpredictability continued in attempts to manage this "invisible enemy." The struggles continued in proving what worked and what did not work in the absence of scientific results from randomized clinical studies. In the beginning, like the majority of general practitioners in primary care settings, I abided by the regulations to "stay home to save lives." Yet as I did, an intense battle erupted inside my mind and heart. I felt overwhelmed by compassion for helping victims; in primary care we could have prevented this disaster from spreading as far and wide as it did.

Practicing telemedicine (common during the pandemic) from my home office, I advised patients if they got sick from COVID-19 and their symptoms worsened, to first call an emergency department to be triaged by well-trained staff. Then, if needed, to call 911 for an evaluation by professionals, per protocol. The 911 staff needed to know that they were presenting with COVID-19 symptoms in order to use personal protective equipment (PPE) and take extra precautions for everyone's safety.

However, this war on the mind started to take its toll. Panic and desperation overwhelmed much of the population as people constantly heard news reports about the virus spreading rapidly among acquaintances, family members, and friends. Whether in their local community or other states and nations, they kept hearing stories about victims being admitted to the hospital and getting placed on ventilators for as long as two or three weeks. This often caused long-term damage to the lungs or other organs. Some died prematurely.

[31] Domenico Cucinotta and Maurizo Vaneli, "WHO Declares COVID-19 a Pandemic," ActaBiomed, March 19, 2020, reprinted by National Center for Biotechnology Information, https://pubmed.ncbi.nlm.nih.gov/32191675/.

A few of our relatives in Europe and some close friends contracted COVID-19 and passed away, leaving all our families with deep emotional pain and psychological trauma. Early in the spring, close relatives told me that an aunt, one brother-in-law's cousin, one niece's brother-in-law, and three close friends between fifty and eighty years of age had passed away in a brief period of time. I had never heard of so many deaths under such conditions. The news that this virus was aggressive and unpredictable proved alarming. It seemed anyone could become a victim at any time.

Then I received calls from our community in northwest Oregon that some of our friends were very sick in the hospital and on a ventilator. Several well-known figures in our community passed away after never receiving early treatment at home. In desperation and terrible distress, sick acquaintances called me, asking about available treatments and what they could do to escape the bad news being disseminated daily by the media. Namely, that early intervention recommended by Frontline Doctors was "misinformation."

Panic Sets In

Patients started to panic when facing the uncomfortable approach recommended by health authorities. They felt pressed to look for solutions in other countries. I realized that many patients from minority groups had resorted to treating themselves at home with medications from foreign countries. Many patients told me that they had started to take medications as soon as they felt sick; some texted me pictures of those medications.

Many were importing medications from outside of the US: Europe, Italy, Russia, Romania, Canada, or Mexico. I heard that some had also brought in medications from Africa. (How ironic, that Americans would reach the point of desperation of seeking help by bringing in medications from underdeveloped nations.) As the media emphasized the subject and disseminated information about the numbers of deaths rising rapidly, these reports scared people to death. To save their lives, they literally took matters into their own hands.

When the Oregon nursing board investigated, they accused me of giving people medications from other countries, but that wasn't true. I had no control over people's private lives, especially those who bypassed primary care settings. Abject fear of the pandemic spurred people to self-medicate. They did so in spite of our clinic's strong emphasis: DO NOT TAKE any medication without medical professionals' advice. Privately, I wondered: How can this be happening in the world's most developed nation, in the most advanced civilization, and with the most qualified experts in the world?

My instincts told me that something was not right in medicine. Not when patients couldn't find any solutions during the most stressful time of their lives. They found no help from the medical community and primary care practices—the very places where they are supposed to get their first interventions for wellbeing and to prevent sickness and hospitalization. That is because there were no ethics in medicine at this point. None whatsoever. People needed to find solutions for their health to save their own lives.

I ask the same question I did at the end of chapter 2: What's wrong with this picture?

Chapter 9

Turning to Telemedicine

In their quest to save their own lives, people turned to telemedicine online, searching for treatments and solutions from pharmacies in other states and even other nations. The majority of US pharmacies were not allowed to honor doctors' orders and prescriptions to provide "off-label" treatment during the most needed time. The situation reminded me of the admonition the angels gave to Lot: "Escape for your life! Do not look behind you nor stay anywhere in the plain. Escape to the mountains, lest you be destroyed" (Gen. 19:17).

It must have been patients' instincts telling them that they must "escape to the mountains"—in their case, to a different state or foreign country—to get medication so the virus would not destroy them. Another passage of Scripture came to mind as I reflected on people's actions in their desperate situations, seeking wisdom from God so they could treat themselves and their families. The ancient people of Israel who fear the Lord experienced supernatural power and divine protection and divine intervention in their lives. This happened during another form of pandemic created by Pharaoh, the powerful ruler of Egypt:

"The king of Egypt said to the Hebrew midwives, whose names were Shiphrah and Puah, 'When you are helping the Hebrew women during childbirth on the delivery stool, if you see that the baby is a boy, kill him; but if it is a girl, let her live.' The midwives, however, feared God and did not do what the king of Egypt had told them to do; they let the boys live. Then the king of Egypt summoned the midwives and asked them, 'Why have you done this? Why have you let the boys live?' The midwives answered Pharaoh, 'Hebrew women are not like

Egyptian women; they are vigorous and give birth before the midwives arrive.' So God was kind to the midwives and the people increased and became even more numerous. And because the midwives feared God, he gave them families of their own" (Ex. 1:15–21 NIV).

Reflecting on the story of the Israelis taking action to save their baby boys' lives, I realized that history repeats itself. People who were super-vigilant and treated themselves before arriving at a primary care office or the ER did not die from coronavirus.

The "Shadow of Death"

I saw another parallel to Scripture at work in the stories of patients who told me that they went through a brush with death. One particular patient, R (dear to our family), told me: "I saw death with my own eyes last night." R's symptoms from COVID-19 got worse at home without early intervention. I cannot imagine how stressful and fearful it must be to be close to dying and yet be alert, all the time knowing that you are on death's doorstep. Another patient who was very sick from the virus told me he felt "like dying" during the night, and that he feared he "would not last until morning." But he prayed and trusted the Lord through all the pain and suffering, and God spared my patient's life.

Hearing such stories made Psalm 23:4 take on a new reality and perspective for me: "Yea, though I walk through the valley of the shadow of death, I will fear no evil: for thou art with me; thy rod and thy staff they comfort me" (KJV). This verse often came to mind during those days. The truth of Scripture was often the only hope I could offer in the moments after I insisted a patient needed to call 911 immediately but they refused. As much as I tried to persuade seriously ill patients to go to the hospital, nearly all of them wanted to prevent that from occurring.

In those conditions, I wanted to do whatever it took to save someone's life. Physicians and nurse practitioners are thinking about the highest authority to guide us in making decisions on how to treat patients who fear death. I also looked up to the Highest Authority, who made me feel those patients' pain during the darkest moment of their life. God guided me to make decisions to help them in their most critical moment, with the best of medicine and the best of Christ. I felt that I walked with every patients through the most fear-inducing and painful moments of their lives.

Do No Harm

Guiding my thoughts throughout these traumatic months was the dictate founded in the legendary Hippocratic Oath that has guided the medical community for more than 2,500 years: "Do no harm." And, to do good to those around me. The damage and devastation that crippled sick people infected with the lethal pathogen made me feel so uncomfortable, that our clinic couldn't adhere to the directions from the authorities to do nothing. So, at the risk of losing my license I started to save lives with early interventions. As I worked, the Bible verse that guided me came from 2 Samuel: "And now may the LORD show kindness and truth to you. I also will repay you this kindness, because you have done this thing" (2 Sam. 1:6).

The suffering patients crying out for help forced me out of my comfort zone. Patients have the right to early treatment. Denying treatment was an infringement of those rights. My first thought was to do no harm to patients came when I prescribed early treatments. Since the virus led down the path of destruction, any little early interventions made a huge difference. As I reflected on the goodness of God in my life, I couldn't stay idle, careless, or impassive. I couldn't let patients' health deteriorate and deliver them a death sentence.

Showing kindness early in the pandemic was crucial. I was shocked when almost all pharmacies said that they could not fill prescriptions for HCQ for patients with COVID-19. They said if they filled off-label prescriptions for people with COVID-19, they would not have adequate supplies for patients who had used this medication for years for rheumatoid arthritis (RA), lupus, or other conditions.

That raised a serious question in my mind: Why couldn't we be kind and give ten tablets of HCQ as a short-term treatment for five days? A vital treatment for a distressed person with viral symptoms, along with other medications, could prevent hospitalization. By comparison, other patients with RA or lupus take about 730 tablets per year. Could these patients who had taken this medication for so many years use different alternatives to address their conditions? Especially in light of the fact that rheumatologists now have more options then HCQ to treat RA, lupus, and other illnesses.

Even though we do not all share the same vision in our practice—whether that involves medicine, expertise, profession, or politics—when so many people's lives are badly affected by a deadly virus that puts them at risk of rapid deterioration and death, we must act with kindness, even if it involves our enemy. As Christ said in His legendary "Sermon on the Mount": "But love your enemies, do good, and lend, hoping for nothing in return; and your reward will be great, and you will be sons of the Most High. For He is kind to the unthankful and evil" (Luke 6:35).

Providing a Solution

The president of the US was willing to share publicly and was not ashamed to tell the world that he was taking an anti-malaria drug to prevent COVID-19. We should have rejoiced and embraced that solution (not criticize) until we had scientific data to prove what would work and what would not work. Instead of rejoicing over President Trump's statement, the "experts" and mainstream media acted outrageously, launching a verbal war against this proposal on every channel far and wide and on social media, placing the entire population in terrible distress. While the "experts" said no solution existed, that wasn't true. I believe President Trump's heroic act to share with the nation saved countless lives, including mine and my family's.

But don't just take my word for it. Earlier I cited a study written by Dr. Peter McCullough and a team of twenty other physicians. In a feature story about McCullough's battle with the virus, journalist Mary Beth Pfeiffer wrote: "When the history of COVID is written, McCullough said, it will be 'very unkind' to those who crafted a paradigm that withheld treatment until patients were so debilitated that hospitalization was needed. The National Institutes of Health will be called to account. 'It didn't do a single clinical trial for patients at home for COVID-19, not a single one,' McCullough told me."[32]

In another part of Pfeiffer's article, she wrote: "'We cannot have patients at risk, like myself, sit at home with no treatment,' McCullough said. ... 'It's wrong and it shouldn't happen.' Sick with COVID and showing signs of respiratory distress, McCullough continued his crusade two days later, posting a YouTube video on why the hospital-dependent approach must change. In Italy, he said, 12 percent of hospital patients on oxygen succumb to COVID, as do 22 to 34 percent of Americans who land in the ICU. 'All of this,' he commented, 'in my view is largely avoidable.'"[33]

In chapter 4, I mentioned how the study led by McCullough talked about the necessity of early interventions for COVID-19 patients to prevent hospitalization: "A low dose of well-known hydroxychloroquine is recommended in the algorithm with other well-known medications to treat early COVID-19 symptoms for outpatients' early management."[34] These are respected physicians and doctors' findings, not the "quacks" portrayed in so many medical circles and news media reports.

Our Greatest Enemy

Fear is the greatest enemy to our immune system, a fact rooted in biblical truth. In my talk at the Romanian Parliament, I quoted 1 John

[32] Mary Beth Pfeiffer, "This Doctor has COVID. He has a plan. For all of us." *TrialSite News*, October 30, 2020, https://vivelifecenter.com/wp-content/uploads/2020/11/This-Doctor-has-COVID.pdf.

[33] Ibid.

[34] "Pathophysiological Basis and Rationale for Early Outpatient Treatment of SARS-CoV-2 (COVID-19) Infection."

4:18: "There is no fear in love; but perfect love casts out fear, because fear involves torment. But he who fears has not been made perfect in love." To that I would add verses 19–20: "We love Him because He first loved us. If someone says, 'I love God,' and hates his brother, he is a liar; for he who does not love his brother whom he has seen, how can he love God whom he has not seen?"

Fear is the greatest enemy to our immune system but love casts out fear, even in medicine. During the pandemic (especially lockdowns), fear became a psychological bioterrorist weapon. When the news spread in the first few months that people were dying by the thousands daily in other countries, fear gripped people's hearts. I knew what that implied. I have spent more than three decades providing end-of-life care to dying people in long-term settings. As I mentioned earlier, I have seen thousands of dying patients while providing palliative care at their bedside during their last days of life. I know well what the dying process looks like and the devastating emotions of anxiety, depression, and despair caused by death.

The year 2020 represented the worst of times. Patients were suffering, their families were desperate, and professional people were helpless and hopeless in the face of death. Everybody is devastated by the dying process, especially when it is as unexpected as it was from COVID-19. Even today, families are still grieving their loved ones who died prematurely. I still mourn the loss of relatives and good friends in our community.

With all the restrictions of the pandemic, we had to treat all manner of illnesses and diseases—not just COVID-19—via telemedicine. Driven by my burning desire to see patients healed, I constantly wondered why we couldn't treat patients with serious symptoms earlier at home. Numerous patients asked me that question. The "why? why? why?" questions still echo through my mind. We will probably never know the full answer.

Not only did that stir my compassion, it made me dwell more about the question of why we were waiting for people to get sick enough with severe symptoms and deteriorate before our own eyes. To get so sick they would have to go to the emergency room, terrified that they would be admitted to the hospital for more aggressive interventions that may work or not. And, that they would end up with post-COVID-19 damage. (More about that later.) Why could we not start that treatment earlier and prevent all the unnecessary turmoil?

As I mentioned in chapter 4, the lack of randomized, controlled trials severely hampered the medical response to the virus outbreak. Such trials need several years, but during the pandemic we did not have time to wait. Time was precious and to save lives we could have used more common sense and experience in the medical field.

The Lord Speaks

God speaks to us through His Word when we listen. One day as I contemplated the terrible situation in primary care management, the Holy Spirit brought to mind a story from 2 Kings. Four leprous men realized that if they sat and did nothing during a time of famine, they would die. If they went into city where famine also reigned, they would likely die there. So they might as well surrender to the enemy. While that might have seemed foolish, God spared their lives because they decided to "do something" about the situation:

"Now there were four leprous men at the entrance of the gate; and they said to one another, 'Why are we sitting here until we die? If we say, "We will enter the city," the famine is in the city, and we shall die there. And if we sit here, we die also. Now therefore, come, let us surrender to the army of the Syrians. If they keep us alive, we shall live; and if they kill us, we shall only die.' And they rose at twilight to go to the camp of the Syrians; and when they had come to the outskirts of the Syrian camp, to their surprise no one was there. For the Lord had caused the army of the Syrians to hear the noise of chariots and the noise of horses—the noise of a great army; so they said to one another, 'Look, the king of Israel has hired against us the kings of the Hittites and the kings of the Egyptians to attack us!'

"Therefore they arose and fled at twilight, and left the camp intact—their tents, their horses, and their donkeys—and they fled for their lives. And when these lepers came to the outskirts of the camp, they went into one tent and ate and drank, and carried from it silver and gold and clothing, and went and hid them; then they came back and entered another tent, and carried some from there also, and went and hid it. Then they said to one another, 'We are not doing right. This day is a day of good news, and we remain silent. If we wait until morning light, some punishment will come upon us. Now therefore, come, let us go and tell the king's household'" (2 Kings 7:1–9).

The four leprous men saved their lives because of their prompt action during crises and a refusal to stay in the same spot, doing nothing during an extreme crisis. As I meditated on this Old Testament story, I asked myself the same question those lepers did: Why should I sit still and do nothing? To watch the news of so many dying around me was devastating. If I did not treat those suffering from this deadly virus, they would die. It would be better to treat them early before their symptoms grew worse.

When I heard during an outbreak in our community many people had contracted the virus and were developing severe symptoms and dying in a matter of weeks, my heart filled with compassion for the victims and their families. My thoughts in my mind went to King Jesus, the Son of God, and what He did when He saw people lacking hope and support: "But when He saw the multitudes, He was moved with compassion for them, because they were weary and scattered, like sheep having no shepherd" (Matt. 9:36).

Reading that verse brought tears to my eyes, knowing that patients infected with the COVID-19 virus were also weary with no hope, weak and lethargic, and sentenced to die. I thought, "If we are in the healing field, why are our hearts not moved with compassion in primary care settings?" It made me so uncomfortable to be a primary care provider, with a mission to help the most vulnerable people with the love of Christ. I could no longer fail to use all my intellectual and material resources, even if it cost me everything I had. Reinforcing my feelings were the words of our Lord: "Blessed are those who are persecuted for righteousness' sake, for theirs is the kingdom of heaven. Blessed are you when they revile and persecute you, and say all kinds of evil against you falsely for My sake. Rejoice and be exceedingly glad, for great is your reward in heaven, for so they persecuted the prophets who were before you" (Matt. 5:10–12).

I might have to wait, but I know the rewards are coming.

Chapter 10

Preventing Hospitalization

My first Covid patient was a friend I will call Lindy. She was working in a community-based care facility as a nurse, caring for elderly patients with multiple chronic conditions. She did not have the typical symptoms, such as increased breathing difficulties; persistent, severe chest pain and pressure; confusion; fatigue; or such severe weakness a patient would struggle to make it to the bathroom. And, since Lindy only had mild Covid symptoms, she could not stay home to wait for her symptoms to get worse until forced to go the hospital. Nor would she think of abandoning her frail, elderly patients.

Lindy's case is a primary reason I acted as I did. I knew I couldn't advise her to stay home and wait for things to get worse, to be followed by a trip to the hospital that could prove fatal. I knew there had to be a better method than the ill-advised "sicken in place" and "hospital dependent" approach. Being around the sick and providing care for dying people for three decades had sharpened my knowledge, given me insights, and made my instincts hypervigilant around sick people.

So, as I mentioned in chapter 2, I started looking for solutions. I diligently searched online for updated information, consulted with experts in infectious diseases, and talked with professionals involved directly in patient care, both in the US and abroad. I asked numerous physicians and health care experts for recommendations for outpatient care for those with COVID-19 symptoms.

Nearly six months into the pandemic, I realized that despite the most advanced medical technology and the best experts in medicine, epidemiology, virology, and pharmaceuticals, we were still struggling with a lack of guidance in primary care. We were failing to help those suffering from such an unpredictable and aggressive virus. I realized how limited we were in the face of this so-rightly named "invisible enemy" that had created panic—a physical, social, economic, and psychological bioterrorist disaster. At this point I decided to listen to my instinct (the still, small voice inside has guided me to solutions in many difficult situations) and common sense to treat patients. I would stand and fight to prevent a terrible event from becoming more disastrous.

I thoroughly reviewed information with the protocol and algorithm published in the Journal of American Medicine to make a well-informed decision. I did this while not knowing that down the road an outbreak of COVID-19 would be waiting to attack our community. More relatives and friends would need my help as a general practitioner and primary care provider to intervene at an early stage to prevent disease, hospitalization, and premature death.

While this can sound simple in retrospect, at the time I battled severe doubts, fear, nervousness over the potential loss of my license, and spiritual foes so nasty they reminded me of the battle Paul warned of: "For we do not wrestle against flesh and blood, but against principalities, against powers, against the rulers of the darkness of this age, against spiritual hosts of wickedness in the heavenly places" (Eph. 6:12).

One day as I pondered this dilemma, I heard a voice so soft it sounded like a whisper: "Choose life solutions with early interventions." Later, I would recognize the parallel to Moses's warning from God to the children of Israel as they were about to cross into the promised land: "I call heaven and earth as witnesses today against you, that I have set before you life and death, blessing and cursing; therefore choose life, that both you and your descendants may live" (Deut. 30:19).

Prevention and Promotion

Early in my medical education, I developed a deep appreciation for disease prevention and health promotion. I liked these courses the most and paid close attention to instruction about what could be done in our society to prevent diseases of any kind and promote health. This prevention and promotion ethic "got into my blood" and became a part of my medical DNA. I wanted to do everything possible to help others understand that prevention is the key to a healthy life, physically and spiritually. (I addressed that subject in my first book, Find Your Peace.)

When diseases from the COVID-19 virus started to appear, I was worried that nothing had been discovered for early interventions for outpatient treatment to prevent hospitalization. There was little aside from over-the-counter medications for low-grade fever, mild to moderate pain, and—to some extent—for coughing. Learning that COVID-19 was so unpredictable and aggressive for those who become infected with a higher viral load, I knew that we needed to also be aggressive with early medical intervention. We needed to use our expertise to prevent further damage to the body. OTC remedies would not be sufficient to treat those in need serious treatment for severe, acute respiratory syndrome coronavirus 2 (SARS-CoV-2).

Most media reports I saw only reviewed hospitals' interventions and mechanical ventilation. Some health authorities proudly told of acquiring thousands of ventilators to prepare for this deadly virus, not knowing that many people died from the wrong protocol with mechanical ventilators. Experts were learning about the pathophysiology of the diseases caused by COVID-19 being an inflammatory disease triggered by the spike protein in the virus that causes "organized pneumonia." This is a rare lung disorder that can cause shortness of breath, cough, weight loss, and wheezing. It is also difficult to treat in late phases.

My heart sank as months went by and no health authorities offered us guidance regarding early interventions for those infected with the virus and too afraid to go to the emergency room, assuming they would be placed on a ventilator and die. I cringed at the toll the virus and the health system's response was creating in our society.

Another victim was a friend I'll call Mia, an active businesswoman who ran a foster care facility, caring for frail elderly people in her home. She enjoyed her work, which included her husband and their only daughter. I had known Mia and her family for more than twenty years. We met often at church and community events, such as weddings, bridal showers, Bible studies, and women's events. She was a beautiful, energetic woman who loved to socialize, sing, pray, and converse with others in the community.

Tragically, Mia was exposed to COVID-19. As soon as she experienced mild symptoms, she went to the emergency room for evaluation and treatment. Instead, a doctor there sent her home and told her to stay there until her symptoms grew worse. The second week of her infection, the symptoms worsened and she went back to the hospital, where a doctor told her, "You came too late." Two days later she died at the relatively young age of fifty-five. Her husband and daughter were stunned. Devastated, he had to close the business, leaving him to deal with two profound losses. He and his daughter are still grieving her loss, as are many in their close-knit immigrant community.

Mia's death reflected what so many of my patients had heard: reports of thousands of people dying in hospitals around the US and other countries, such as Italy and Brazil. And all in a short period of time. Patients expressed their concerns to me over and over again, their hearts gripped by intense fear and panic. According to news reports, the majority of those who were dying were placed on a ventilator as a last resort, but never returned home.

Early Treatment

Each patient who tested positive or developed symptoms when exposed to Covid begged me to help them get treatment as early as possible at home. They didn't want to get within sniffing distance of a hospital. This raised the concern in my mind: Why could we not treat COVID-19 patients at home earlier instead, when the symptoms began? This would prevent panic from fear of hospitals, as well as psychological distress caused by untreated symptoms and thoughts of uncertainty and the unknown.

For close supervision and further complex interventions, we could then send to hospitals only those patients with severe symptoms that could not be treated at home. Doctors and specialists who were working with patients with COVID-19 in the hospital were also terrified by the lack of solutions to save lives. But they realized that they could treat symptoms caused by the virus, based on the pathophysiological response of every system in the body.

Many doctors and specialists posted video clips on social media, circulating useful information about what they had learned during the disease process about the pathophysiology. They told about how they had intervened, based on their knowledge gained over the years about potential medications to save patients' lives. But those video clips with priceless information from doctors and experts around the world were often censored and the clips removed from the public's eyes. This deprived physicians and the general public of information about early treatment that could have saved many lives.

Hospitalists used well-known medications from their accumulated experience of years of daily practice in medicine. Medications used before for different diseases were used now for symptoms of COVID-19 to reduce inoculation. Antiviral therapy, immuno-modulators, and corticosteroids were used to treat the inflammation and micro thrombosis produced by spike protein and debris from inflammation from the cytokine storm caused by the virus.

They began to administer bronchodilators via inhalers or nebulizers, and oxygen supplementation to treat breathing difficulties and the oxygen deficiency known as hypoxia—a condition caused by low oxygen levels—to assist people with breathing. But the good information about early interventions were suppressed by the media and labeled as "misinformation." Doctors who dared to treat patients with early symptoms with off-label and repurposed safe medications were threatened, harassed, and persecuted by health authorities around the world.

Saving Lives

I had no doubt that "care at home" could save lives. I was familiar with this practice because of my years of experience in the long-term care field, when I had to regularly care for acutely and chronically ill people at home. The goal was to keep these frail patients out of the hospital. Professionals had been talking about treatment in the home for decades; house calls and home health practices developed in order to provide care to people in the comfort of their own homes. And, prevent hospitalization.

Many times, we had to provide post-operative care with complex interventions for patients at home, using well-known, complex medications and procedures. Among them were nebulizers and oxygen supplementation for COPD, asthma, and other lung conditions. I was familiar with caring for tracheostomies, colostomies, and ileostomies; using portable ventilators; using complex medications via nasal tubes; catheter care; and treatments for multiple chronic conditions. The latter included a number of medications: antibiotics, antivirals, anti-coagulants, anti-hypertensives, anti-diabetes, and complex pain control measures.

I had thirty years of experience working in long-term care facilities with a home-like environment as a provider, manager, and owner of those facilities. We cared for residents with multiple chronic conditions and treated them with all of the medications that were being used now for patients with COVID-19-linked diseases (except treatment via IV infusion). This opened my eyes to the possibility of treating patients in the community with symptoms from the virus, in the comfort of their own homes.

For example, antibiotics could be used for upper and lower respiratory infections. Anti-inflammatory drugs and corticosteroids were good for patients with inflammation in their lungs that caused wheezing and difficulty breathing. Immunomodulatory drugs, such as hydroxychloroquine (used for more than fifty years for autoimmune diseases with inflammatory processes), had multiple uses. Bronchodilators could treat shortness of breath and offer oxygen supplementation for patients with low oxygen levels from hypoxia. There were also such treatments as antipyretics for high fever, analgesics for pain, and anti-congestion and cough medications for congestion and cough.

I was familiar with all of these medications and procedures for administration. Because of my medical background, I considered it quite possible—and reasonable—to treat patients with symptoms from COVID-19 at home. Not only could these methods be used to treat acute, mild, or moderate symptoms, it would alleviate the fears of suffering patients. As I mentioned in chapter 4, fear affects the immune system in a negative way by aggravating the symptoms from infection, leading to more decline of patients. Patients' quality of life is highly affected without early intervention during a disease's process.

As I contemplated the good that could be done through early interventions, the Holy Spirit was working on my heart. He brought to mind a Bible passage that made me quite uncomfortable about failing to act to help suffering people: "Ask, and it will be given to you; seek, and you will find; knock, and it will be opened to you. For everyone who asks receives, and he who seeks finds, and to him who knocks it will be opened. Or what man is there among you who, if his son asks for bread, will give him a stone? Or if he asks for a fish, will he give him a serpent? If you then, being evil, know how to give good gifts to your children, how much more will your Father who is in heaven give good things to those who ask Him! Therefore, whatever you want men to do to you, do also to them, for this is the Law and the Prophets" (Matt. 7:7–12).

The Holy Spirit was working on my heart and mind to ask, seek, and knock.

Compelled to Act

Compelled by compassion, I decided not to sit and do nothing any longer. To get the ball rolling, I reached out to a doctor and university professor with impeccable credentials to solicit her thoughts on the pandemic. I wanted to know about my options for early interventions at our small clinic. After we talked, I checked a number of her professional postings on social media, which confirmed she was well-informed on scientifically-proven treatment.

During our conversation, she referred me to the algorithm from a study published in The American Journal of Medicine. The "Pathophysiological Basis and Rationale for Early Outpatient Treatment of SARS-CoV-2 (COVID-19) Infection" is the study by Dr. Peter McCullough and a team of twenty other physicians that I mentioned in my talk in Romania (chapter 4). While this opened my eyes to the solution and hope for patients in our community, information about this algorithm was not widely disseminated, which meant we had to struggle with a lack of guidance.

My struggle was with the rules and regulations of the FDA that as providers we must follow, but I learned quickly (as I mentioned in chapter 2) that this agency acknowledges that physicians have the legal right to prescribe already-approved drugs "off label" when they deem that appropriate. The Holy Spirit working inside me led me to intervene at any cost. Without delay, I started treating patients with COVID-19 symptoms.

Once they heard about what we were doing, patients started calling our clinic every day. And why not treat them? For years, those medications had been used for patients with acute and chronic diseases. We had administered them daily in our foster homes and memory care facilities for a variety of illnesses, with no side effects or adverse reactions. One patient called me the third day of her treatment for the COVID-19 virus to say, "I cannot believe what a difference these medications have made for me. I feel like a completely different person. My energy level came back. It is a night-and-day difference."

I had often witnessed firsthand the fear, anxiety, and anguish of people who had tested positive for COVID-19. They were experiencing mild, moderate, or severe symptoms that inflicted scars on their emotional, psychological, and physical well-being. I couldn't wait any longer and let people suffer without early intervention. Especially when we had medications available at an affordable price for patients to treat their symptoms at home. During the many calls we received, I could sense patients' emotional pain and psychological distress. I treated every person like a member of my family—with great responsibility, love, and compassion.

As we continued treating patients, I also searched diligently for published articles in medical journals. I knew we lacked the best evidence, such as randomized, controlled studies that are imperative for gathering evidence of the best practices for caring for COVID-19 patients. But because of the brief time available to obtain such results and collect data to guide our own practice, I considered it imperative to use the knowledge about medications that I had accumulated over the years. To do anything less would have been a dereliction of my duty, even if the state nursing board didn't like it.

Chapter 11

Learning from the President

At the outset of the pandemic, confusion reigned. With a flurry of contradictory reports airing daily, I struggled to find a reliable source for appropriate information. With news channels instilling fear through their largely negative reports, I turned to listening to President Trump and focusing on his heart. As I learned more about the president, I reflected on his statements about the possibility of preventative actions and early interventions with hydroxychloroquine. At the same time, I could not wrap my mind around the unkind decisions to withhold early treatments and interventions. I could not imagine how anyone could suggest we wait for patients to get so sick and debilitated by the COVID-19 virus that they needed hospitalization, intensive care, or mechanical ventilation.

We could have learned from the president's experience with prophylactic treatment and those doctors who had so much expertise in primary care management in treating patients earlier. Treatment that could have prevented so much hospitalization and further damage to millions of patients—physically, emotionally, socially, and economically. In March of 2020 I heard President Trump saying he had used HCQ prophylactically as a preventative measure. Common sense told me that the US president's doctors must be the best in the world and would never prescribe harmful medications to the leader of the free world.

For several years, I had prescribed low doses of hydroxychloroquine for patients with rheumatoid arthritis, lupus, and other multiple chronic diseases. I had even prescribed it prophylactically for malaria for those who traveled to Africa. No one reported any negative side effects. One patient with multiple chronic diseases—such as diabetes, hypertension, and coronary artery disease—took this medication every day for more than ten years. Not only did she never report side effects or adverse reactions, one time she told me: "I feel good."

I also knew that millions around the world used this medication to treat symptoms from viruses on a regular basis, including over-the-counter varieties. For COVID-19 symptoms, protocol for early intervention was a low dose of HCQ for five days, twice a day, or a total of ten tablets (in some cases this could be repeated for five more days). As mentioned earlier, this compares to patients taking thousands of tablets of HCQ for ten to twenty years for rheumatoid arthritis, lupus, and malaria. Some take it throughout their lifetime.

At that time, HCQ worked for the president, quite likely saving his life. The president recognized that there were no randomized, controlled trials or scientific evidence to prove the effectiveness of hydroxychloroquine for COVID-19. At one news briefing he said while there was a lack of scientific evidence, it had worked for him: "It's a very strong, powerful medicine, but it doesn't kill people. You've seen the same test I have. In France, they had a very good test. But we don't have time to go and say, gee, let's take a couple years and test it out. And let's go and test with the test tubes and the laboratories. We don't have time. I'd love to do that."[35]

Previous Evidence

The president was right: during a pandemic there is no time to get results from a randomized, controlled trial for the best evidence practice. Still, there was previous evidence of HCQ's efficacy, dating back to the original outbreak of severe acute respiratory syndrome (SARS) in Guangdong Province, China, in late 2002. An article in the Virology Journal that appeared in 2005 stated that "chloroquine has strong antiviral effects on SARS-CoV infection of primate cells. These

---

[35] Lev Facher, "Fact-checking Trump's claims about hydrochloroquine, the antimalarial drug he's touting as a coronavirus treatment," Stat News, April 6, 2020, https://www.statnews.com/2020/04/06/trump-hydroxychloroquine-fact-check/.

inhibitory effects are observed when the cells are treated with the drug either before or after exposure to the virus, suggesting both prophylactic and therapeutic advantage. In addition to the well-known functions of chloroquine such as elevations of endosomal pH, the drug appears to interfere with terminal glycosylation of the cellular receptor, angiotensin-converting enzyme 2.

"This may negatively influence the virus-receptor binding and abrogate the infection, with further ramifications by the elevation of vesicular pH, resulting in the inhibition of infection and spread of SARS CoV at clinically admissible concentrations. Chloroquine is effective in preventing the spread of SARS CoV in cell culture. Favorable inhibition of virus spread was observed when the cells were either treated with chloroquine prior to or after SARS CoV infection. In addition, the indirect immunofluorescence assay described herein represents a simple and rapid method for screening SARS-CoV antiviral compounds."[36]

Despite such evidence, the news media harshly criticized the president for speaking publicly about taking this medication prophylactically. The negative tone of so much media coverage of the president's stance was a major disservice to the public. I saw little reason to criticize the president for taking a prudent measure to prolong his life during such a crucial time. Many publications made untrue statements about HCQ being "unproven" when it was a well-tested medication, one used by millions around the globe for more than five decades. True, it was used off-label, but the truth is many other drugs are prescribed routinely by medical professionals to treat symptoms from illnesses caused by viruses, bacteria, and other diseases. President Trump relied on the best information his doctors and other medical experts provided him—and prescribed for him. That was a clue for other people to do the same as a life-saving measure.

---

[36] Martin J. Vincent, Eric Bergeron, et. al., "Chloroquine is a potent inhibitor of SARS coronavirus infection and spread," Virology Journal 2, article 69, August 22, 2005, https://virologyj.biomedcentral.com/articles/10.1186/1743-422X-2-69.

Not surprisingly, by that July the BBC reported that demand for hydroxychloroquine had increased, with widespread interest in it as both a preventative measure and for treating patients with coronavirus. In fact, at that time there were more than two hundred trials underway worldwide on HCQ's impact, either as a prophylactic or treatment for COVID-19.

"Promotion by leading political figures such as President Trump has led to both hydroxychloroquine, and the related drug chloroquine, becoming the subject of widespread speculation online about their potential benefits and harmful effects," the BBC reported. "This has led to high demand for the drugs and global supply shortages. There's also been controversy within the scientific community.

"Trials around the world were temporarily derailed when a study published in The Lancet claimed the drug increased fatalities and heart problems in some patients. The results prompted the World Health Organization (WHO) and others to halt trials over safety concerns. However, the Lancet subsequently retracted the study when it was found to have serious shortcomings and the WHO resumed its trials."[37]

There were many doctors with decades of experience in medicine from whom we could learn about the best approach to fighting COVID-19 when no scientific evidence from randomized, controlled trials existed. The fact that they caught the attention of the president did not surprise me. Nor did his willingness to alert the public, a fact that brought to mind the statement Jesus made on His triumphal entry into Jerusalem. When the Pharisees complained about His disciples praising and glorifying Him, Christ said: "I tell you that if these should keep silent, the stones would immediately cry out" (Luke 19:40).

---

[37] Jack Goodman and Christopher Giles, "Coronavirus and hydroxychloroquine: What do we know?" BBC, July 27, 2020, https://www.bbc.com/news/51980731.

Speaking Up

President Trump did not keep silent, crying out to the American people and the world that there was hope through his disclosure that he was taking HCQ. He encouraged the American people—who were rightly scared by this unpredictable, aggressive virus—to take it prophylactically as he did. He was right in presenting HCQ as being an antidote for COVID-19 for the majority of people if taken early, before their symptoms worsened.

Indeed, less than nine months after I heard of President Trump taking HCQ, a report appeared in the Washington Examiner about a peer-reviewed study that determined low-dose hydroxy-chloroquine, combined with zinc and azithromycin, was an effective therapeutic approach against COVID-19. The story noted that HCQ became a controversial issue at the height of the pandemic when Trump championed it as an effective treatment, drawing criticism from the media and several health experts. I found it highly significant that Twitter (now X) censored a video that summer showing doctors touting the drug's effectiveness.

"A total of 141 patients diagnosed with the coronavirus were treated with the three-drug cocktail over a period of five days and compared to a control group of 377 people who tested positive for the virus but were not given the treatment," reporter Andrew Mark Miller wrote.

"The study found that 'the odds of (hospitalization) of treated patients was 84 (percent) less than in the untreated patients,' and only one patient died from the group being treated with the drugs compared to 13 deaths in the untreated group. ... Additionally, a July study conducted by the Henry Ford Health System in Michigan concluded that patients taking hydroxychloroquine were more likely to survive the coronavirus."[38]

---

[38] Andrew Mark Miller, "Study finds 84% fewer hospitalizations for patients treated with controversial drug hydroxychloroquine," Washington Examiner, November 25, 2020, https://www.washingtonexaminer.com/news/840424/study-finds-84-fewer-hospitalizations-for-patients-treated-with-controversial-drug-hydroxychloroquine/.

The point here is that much of the media tried to silence the president with their unkind, negative reports and criticism, leaving many citizens tormented by fear. "The stones will cry out" for those who were not treated with early interventions prophylactically and died unnecessarily.

Yet anyone who had the courage to say anything that deviated in the slightest from acceptable health guidance found themselves mocked and ridiculed.

A prime example is Dr. Simone Gold and a team of prominent physicians who spoke (on a video viewed by millions) about using HCQ for patients in the early phase of viral infection, with promising results. Through censorship, the media removed the information from their platforms, stating that they spread "misinformation." Noted one report: "The video was retweeted by President Donald Trump and his son, Donald Trump Jr., and spread like wildfire online, garnering millions of views before it was removed by Facebook, Twitter and YouTube for what the social media companies said was spreading misinformation about the coronavirus."[39]

Calling a low-dose, five-day HCQ treatment "misinformation" is outrageous. Especially when so many states have legalized drugs such as marijuana, which hold multiple adverse consequences over the long term. Abusing this so-called "harmless" substance can lead to neurocognitive syndromes, psychosis, and anti-motivation conditions in young people. Many become homeless and wind up living in miserable conditions—in tattered tents worse than in a third-world environment, with no water to wash their hands.

Such practices put other people in the community at high risk for transmitting infections due to their poor hygiene, no bathrooms, no shower, no laundry, and no civilized conditions. Yet I rarely hear words of criticism on TV or social media platforms about all the bad

---

[39] Stacey Shepard, "Local doctors featured in video that was banned from social media," The Bakersfield Californian, August 9, 2020, https://www.bakersfield.com/news/local-doctorsfeatured-in-viral-video-of-doctors-that-was-laterbanned-from-social-media/article_fd9da404-d8ec11ea-aeae-47e7e993c84d.html.

consequences of legalized marijuana, especially for those younger people who are often destroying their future.

Taking Action

This dichotomy between truth and fiction prompted Dr. Brian Tyson of El Centro, California, to act. He ultimately wound up saving some twenty thousand lives because of prescribing early treatment for coronavirus victims. A veteran of ER and hospital medicine for more than fourteen years, he wrote a first-person account about the craziness of being told to stop prescribing HCQ a month after lockdowns began because it would prohibit hospitals from getting it for those who needed it.

"For the first time in my life as a physician, I was being told to stop saving people's lives!" he wrote. "My response was clear, 'Give me an alternative, and I will use it; until then, I will use whatever I have that has been shown to work.' I have never understood the pushback on using treatments that were maybe controversial but showed promise over the ridiculous policy of 'home quarantine for 14 days' without any treatment. Who does that? Since when is any disease treated by quarantine alone?"[40]

Later, he traveled to Washington, DC to speak at the Supreme Court, a process he called "intimidating" because of the highly intelligent physicians, scholars, lawyers, and researchers who had been invited. Yet, he pressed on, saying his speech came from overcoming fear after treating the multitude of COVID-19 patients who had survived: the students, the staff members, two of his nurse practitioners, both his sons, and his manager's mother. He started by declaring that we could go back to school, to work, and to life because we would not let fear take our freedom any longer.

---

[40] "The miracle of the Imperial Valley: Dr. Tyson's first-person account of COVID-19," The Desert Review, November 1, 2020 (updated April 16, 2021), https://www.thedesertreview.com/news/the-miracle-of-the-imperial-valley-dr-tyson-s-first-person-account-of-covid-19/article_a8707136-196b-11eb-bc7b-87d7730460bb.html.

Tyson said that was a moment he will never forget. Knowing his grandfathers had served in World War II, Korea, and Vietnam, he said he had always wanted to do something great for his country. He talked of his grandfather and father serving in war and how scared they must have been. The fight with COVID-19 was his war, he said, and it wasn't over.

"We are still fighting the fight, and we will continue to do so," he said in his speech. "I hoped the video would be a tool that other physicians could see and hear. We need everyone to see the success we had. When it was finally posted on YouTube, it was exciting—it started to go viral, and then something happened. It was taken down! Why? Why would you take down a video with the knowledge, research, links, and website, where everyone can see what we are doing? Why? I don't have any reason.

"I can't believe that big tech and government controls want to see people die. Why would you take down the message of hope? Why would you take down the message of treatment? Why do you want to continue living in fear, when there are clear treatment options now? There are multiple options. ... That should upset people all over the world. Think about it—the world is looking to us to find a treatment or a cure, and when we do, it gets taken down? ...I was able to get raw video, and we published it again and again. We will keep publishing it over and over, until it is recognized all over the world that we don't need to be afraid anymore. People need to know that we will survive this pandemic, just like those of the past. There is treatment available. It works when used early, and it is very effective."[41]

I could hear in Dr. Tyson's tone of voice that day his compassion for suffering patients to get treated early, with the best we have available in medicine. I sensed the passion in his heart for the world to instill hope in people's minds and to alleviate the crushing fear COVID-19 had inflicted on millions. I also heard his intense agony and

---

[41] The miracle of the Imperial Valley: Dr. Tyson's first-person account of COVID-19."

disappointment over the media's actions to fight against disseminating the information that could bring a ray of hope. As he saw it, the media were depriving the world of a solution that could stop the pandemic with its catastrophic loss of life, leaving nations with damage economically, financially, socially, mentally, and emotionally—for generations to come.

If any crimes were committed during the pandemic, the list should start there.

Chapter 12

The Highest Authority

When people faced an increased risk of losing their lives and health authorities told primary care practitioners to send people home to "sit" on a deadly virus with no early treatment, I had to look to the Highest Authority to determine a proper course of action. I knew that both science and faith were gifts from God, and that we had to use spiritual weapons to wage the battle before us. As Paul wrote, "For the weapons of our warfare are not carnal but mighty in God for pulling down strongholds, casting down arguments and every high thing that exalts itself against the knowledge of God, bringing every thought into captivity to the obedience of Christ" (2 Cor. 10:4–5).

While many ignored this war, we were fighting a merciless, invisible enemy in the form of a lethal pathogen. Then there were the negative news media reports about treatments for COVID-19, as well as actions taken to intimidate hard-working medical practitioners trying to save people's lives. Not many doctors will openly discuss it, but during the pandemic a wave of fear rippled across the medical community. It came in the form of threats to revoke the licenses of anyone who didn't bow down to health or government authorities in all matters related to coronavirus.

But in working to prevent hospitalization and premature death, I had to make life-and-death decisions when providing care to patients suffering from COVID-19-linked diseases. In all my treatment of patients during the pandemic—not only from physical pain, sickness, and disease, but great psychological distress—I needed to obey the

Lord who created science. I had to follow the One who gives faith as a gift that has always guided me when I need direction.

God uses human brains as instruments to manifest His supernatural intelligence to create new advances in medicine, technology, and other frontiers. But those who do not fear God do not give God credit for His investment in humankind's minds. I saw this while living under an immoral communist regime for about three decades. As a person of faith, I gained experience in how to cope with uncertainty in a place where cruel communist leaders with no fear of God governed the nation. They dictated how we were to live our daily lives during various crises, yet without offering us any hope. This created more confusion and oppression—just when life hurt the most. When I faced difficulties and persecution for my values and beliefs, I learned that God is the Highest Authority. I learned that I needed to trust God's Word and run under His mighty wings for divine protection.

In every circumstance, I needed to look up at the Highest Authority that gave me direction and guidance in every step I had to take. The living Word of God has the same sovereign supernatural power today, for every person who believes in God and for those who do not. As David wrote in the Psalms: "From the end of the earth I will cry to You, when my heart is overwhelmed; lead me to the rock that is higher than I" (Ps. 61:2).

Withholding Treatment

As many compassionate doctors did, deep in my heart I asked why the authorities were withholding effective early treatment. Just as the president wondered why we did not want to use early interventions for COVID-19 patients, Dr. Peter McCullough noticed the unkindness of professional primary care practitioners and politicians who were ascending above authentic medical experts in medicine. In his book on the impact of coronavirus on the 2020 election, bestselling author Stephen Strang (once named by Time magazine as one of the nation's twenty-five most influential evangelicals) remarked on the cruelty of withholding early treatment for patients suffering from this aggressive, unpredictable virus.

"They even referred to the treatment as 'snake oil,' even though several studies and medical journals from France, Italy, and China show promising and effective results," Strang wrote in God, Trump, and COVID-19. "Meanwhile, India and other countries limited hydroxychloroquine from being sent out of their countries to other countries. President Trump eventually worked hard to construct a deal with both India and Israel to have millions of doses sent to the United States. It seems the polarization of the American political climate has hit new levels, as even in a pandemic situation there can't seem to be agreement on getting fast and effective medication help to the people."[42]

The same question echoed through my mind: "Why in primary care are we withholding early treatment and waiting for people to 'sicken-in-place,' living in fear of dying from those symptoms that are worsening as time passes, and causing terrible distress physically and emotionally so that they will have no choice but hospitalization?"

I felt desperate to save people's lives in our community so they would not be overwhelmed by fear and despair. God gave me an experience in my practice with multiple patients experiencing signs and symptoms of COVID-19 in different stages, and I observed firsthand their quick recovery with early treatment. I also saw very slow recovery—even hospitalization with lung damage—by patients whose symptoms were not treated early when they were infected. Those who started treatment late in the course of their illness needed hospitalization and mechanical ventilation. Some died prematurely. What a tragedy in the history of twenty-first century medicine!

Saving Lives

One morning my telephone rang. When I answered, a weak voice at the other end told of having a dream that I could help her with her

---

[42] God, Trump, and COVID-19: How the Pandemic is Affecting Christians, the World, and America's 2020 Election, 64.

desperate need for treatment of her terrible symptoms and those of family members. That left me speechless. I realized how God cared for His children by moving in my heart to seek solutions for the helpless people He loves. He even gave them dreams about where to go for help during an outbreak in our community because of the ban on doctors prescribing early treatment.

The pastor of a Romanian church bravely announced from the pulpit that there was hope through our small clinic. He told people they could get help if they were sickened by the virus. After that, many patients called for early interventions, especially after a viral outbreak that followed. Hundreds of patients and their families and close friends pleaded for help after many providers refused to treat COVID-19 symptoms at home. The callers included many pastors and church leaders from our area, whose lives have been saved with early inventions from our small clinic.

Each patient with COVID-19 had a unique clinical presentation of their symptoms. But all reported at least five mild-to-moderate symptoms in the first week; among them were sore throat, dry cough, shortness of breath, fever, headaches, dizziness, or nausea. They reported using over-the-counter preparations for fever, pain, and cough. While they saw some mild results from OTC substances, the symptoms did not go away. The longer they waited, the worse the symptoms grew. Patients started to experience more compulsive coughing, lung congestion, shortness of breath, severe weakness, lethargy, increased fatigue, persistent fever, and other signs. Many panicked as time passed and their health deteriorated.

Severe cases led to more anxiety and psychological distress. The worst-case scenario was when a patient's fever increased to more than 101 degrees Fahrenheit and would not cease (after taking Tylenol and ibuprofen regularly for ten days), and oxygen levels started to drop below 89 percent. This even after using an in-home nebulizer or oxygen supplementation. That was the time when as a care provider I remained on alert and monitored every patient closely as their symptoms progressed. If the patient's condition declined further, I sent them to the hospital for more advanced and aggressive interventions. When people waited too long and symptoms got worse, we could recognize who would live and who would die as a consequence of late intervention.

When their oxygen levels started to drop below 89 percent, patients coughed more and experienced shortness of breath, showing signs of developing life-threatening "organized pneumonia." This was because of the inflammation process caused by the cytokine storm at the alveoli (tiny air sacs in the lungs) level. This is created by the immune system when fighting the COVID-19 virus, which further caused microthrombosis and abnormal blood clots in the lungs' blood vessels, developing into acute respiratory distress syndrome (ARDS). These patients needed to go to the hospital right away for close monitoring and advanced interventions.

But with early outpatient interventions, I helped hundreds of patients to prevent them from contracting organized pneumonia from Covid. (Different from other kinds, organized pneumonia leaves victims with lung damage.) Thus, they were able to recover at home from COVID-19 as from a flu-like illness but more aggressive. Some patients later told of their symptoms improving in two to four days. It was satisfying to see the results of early interventions in mild and moderate COVID-19 symptoms that prevented hospitalization and all its consequences.

Psychological Distress

However, many patients and their families suffered profound psychological distress when their primary care providers refused early interventions. One of these patients whom I will call Joe tested positive for COVID-19. He went to a primary care provider, who instructed him to "isolate at home and to wait for the symptoms to aggravate and only then call a doctor." In the meantime, the doctor told him to drink tea with honey and to take Tylenol or other OTC cold medications. Joe's anxiety increased dramatically. He knew from close friends that the symptoms could aggravate quickly with no intervention. Some wound up in the hospital; a few were placed on a ventilator, and some of them passed away.

Another patient I will call Covey had a compulsive cough and shortness of breath. Her oxygen saturation dropped to 90 percent overnight after eight days of mild symptoms from the virus. Doctors told her that she needed a chest X-ray first to see if she needed treatment. This patient was desperate because there was no place to go to get such a test done. "Nobody wanted to do a chest X-ray for me, until I got out of fourteen days of quarantine," she told me.

She had tested positive for COVID-19 and needed to wait two weeks in quarantine. Not wanting to go to the ER when she was so sick, Covey panicked. Like many patients, nothing else mattered to her when she couldn't breathe. She was in day eight after her symptoms began to manifest. They were worsening instead of getting better. This stemmed from the disease process when the spike protein escapes from cells after multiplying inside the cell. This triggered the immune system to overreact and cause massive inflammation in her body. Especially in the lungs, the site of the highest concentration of the angiotensin converting enzymes 2 receptors and leading to SARS-2.

Covey tried to treat herself with home remedies and OTC preparations, with no results. Her symptoms grew worse by the day. She needed empirical interventions and more aggressive interventions right away at home. When she reported that her oxygen had dropped to 90 percent, I knew that the inflammatory process in her lungs was getting worse. This can cause damage and shortness of breath, wheezing, and difficult breathing. I strongly advised her to go to the emergency room for further evaluation and intervention; her symptoms were consistent with viral pneumonia from COVID-19.

Having little children at home, Covey did not want to go to the hospital. She had heard from news media reports that people who went to the hospital with aggravated symptoms often ended up on a mechanical ventilator. Some did not recover. In fact, just a few weeks earlier in our community, a friend in her mid-fifties had gone to the hospital and was told that she had waited too long and passed away in the hospital. People generally do not know how to assess themselves in order to go to the ER at the right time (nobody does). But I was able to treat symptoms and diseases more aggressively at home in order to prevent hospitalization. This was true even in cases with more severe symptoms. That is, when the patients complied with strict treatment guidelines, close monitoring, and medical supervision.

Fortunately, I was able to successfully treat Covey's illness, but it took longer for her to recover because she had waited so long to ask for help. Her children had to help her with daily activities because she deteriorated day after day due to lack of early treatment. Covey became so lethargic she was able barely able to stand up to go the bathroom. As soon as she started treatment, she started to feel better. While it took a while, she fully recovered with much support from family, friends, and professional physicians. All without hospitalization. (You will read more stories like Covey's in the next chapter.)

Those who sought help earlier—as soon as their symptoms surfaced—received treatment per the algorithm created by Dr. Peter McCullough and other doctors presented earlier for COVID-19. It was based on their clinical presentation and a positive coronavirus test. We followed each patient closely with daily phone calls (some twice a day); according to their reports, their condition improved day by day. They reported that in two to four days their fever had gone down and their oxygen levels went up. They coughed less, their muscle pain and headaches improved, and they started to get up and move around for the activities of daily living. All these improvements came from early interventions.

I have to ask: does this sound to you like "misinformation" or disregard for patients' health? Or was it the health authorities who misled millions of citizens who should have their licenses revoked?

Chapter 13

Restoration Stories

"For if you remain completely silent at this time, relief and deliverance will arise for the Jews from another place, but you and your father's house will perish. Yet who knows whether you have come to the kingdom for such a time as this?" (Est. 4:14).

When the COVID-19 outbreak unleashed its terrible damage on our community, the thought of keeping silent touched off an internal mental struggle. I was terrified at the thought of remaining silent, but equally frightened by the prospect of speaking out and facing intense opposition from those who held the power over my right to practice medicine. As this struggle raged on, the thought went through my mind: "Whose voice do you follow: the voice of intimidation or the voice of those desperate for help?"

Immediately I recognized the voice of intimidation. The same voice as the communist regime I fought more than four decades ago: "You are about to lose your job if the communists find out that you are a person of faith in Christ Jesus, that you believe in the Word of God, that you go to church, or that you go to prayer groups or Bible study..."

I had to make the right decision now. The same one I made four decades ago in the communist country where I lived before arriving in the US: to obey the voice of the Lord. To resolve the issue of this "mind war," I focused on what I knew: all of the medications I prescribed were approved for human use; they had been used for many years and were safe. And now I could use them off-label to save lives.

Ultimately, the voice of the Spirit proved stronger. He persisted and reminded me: "If you remain completely silent at this time, relief and deliverance for the sick people and their diseases will come from other places. But you will be held accountable for not listening to their cries of desperation because you did not help them at such a time as this." After my early and at-home interventions, patients started sending text messages, telling me how good they felt after they started these treatments. So, I asked many of them to write an account of their experiences. I am including just a select number to encourage those who still live with crippling fear of COVID-19 symptoms and the diseases caused by the virus. And some of them mentioned exactly the words from Esther; patient R wrote, "Thank you, Dr. Rodica, for your huge care and love, and for agreeing to be an Esther for such a time like this! You will have a big reward in heaven! Blessings & prayers!"

The board that persecuted me by taking my license away and humiliated me by stating publicly that I was practicing unsafe medicine ignored patients' powerful testimonies of recovery through early interventions and their subsequent healing from symptoms of this deadly virus. Based on their statements, nobody can say: "Frontline Doctors spread misinformation." These stories contain facts and discuss the results of how our actions saved lives through early treatment. Some of the following messages were addressed to me and others to the state nursing board. Their testimonies matter, which is why I am including some of them here.

First-Person Accounts

IR's testimony:

Dear Provider,

My name is IR, daughter of LR, who recently received amazing care. I would like to thank you most profoundly for your diligent and godly care for my mother, and for the hope of healing that came through your clinic! A special thank you to Dr. Rodica Malos. My mother had started showing signs of COVID-19 sometime in early

September: cough, fatigue, diarrhea, loss of taste and smell, and low-grade fever (100.1 to 101).

She managed okay for a week, but her condition deteriorated quickly, to the point where she was very weak and could barely get out of bed. She was breathing heavier, with loss of appetite. We did the best we could for our mother; we encouraged her to take fluids hourly, along with food and rest. It helped, but not nearly enough; she could get up, but weakness was still there. Knowing of Dr. Rodica Malos, I reached out to her to have my mother talk with her in Romanian. Based on that phone call evaluation, she received additional treatment with azithromycin, prednisone, and hydroxychloroquine.

Within a few days of this treatment, my mother's condition and symptoms improved beyond belief! If I recall correctly, within three days of this treatment and the inhaler she was able to make soup for herself and her family that lives with her, and even encourage us with her positive spirit. Praise God! Her breathing became lighter; cough subsided but contained phlegm; her fever dissipated drastically; by the end of the week, she had a normal temperature with no fever-reducing drugs. Her appetite improved so much that she craved certain salads she made with fresh veggies from her garden.

How wonderful is this? What joy came over our family. We felt the spirit of stress and uncertainty flee from our home when Mom came out of the dark hour! I know that in these challenging times, certain treatments these days are undermined if not restricted; I hope and pray that through this letter of encouragement and gratitude you will remain steadfast on the path of good health and support of those suffering.

With warmth and gratefulness on the behalf of LR, IR

V and R's testimony:

Dear Dr. Rodica Malos,

We can't find the words to express our thankfulness to God, Dr. Malos. The HCQ treatment worked right away. Even though my husband has problems with his heart, it is unbelievable. No side effects, just healing and comfort right away. Even after the first tablet we felt the difference. To God be the glory! We are both well. We can enjoy our grandchildren and live a normal, blessed life. And this is just because we have doctors brave enough and who really care about people, no matter how much pressure they have. May God bless Dr. Rodica Malos, who is a wonderful, kind, and very caring person. Please keep doing what you are doing. You save lots of lives. Thank you!

A's testimony:

Hello, this is A, and through this testimony I want to encourage others that were affected by COVID-19 that there is hope. On the week of August 23-29, 2020, I had symptoms of fever on and off; I thought I had a cold, but after that week, on September 1 I felt very weak, and called for an appointment with Dr. Rodica Malos. Afterwards, she prescribed me medication and prayed for me. After the second day of treatment, I had no more fever and my strength started to come back. My oxygen came back to normal and in five days I completed the treatment and fully recovered. Personally, I'm very thankful to God for your clinic and for Dr. Rodica Malos. Keep up the good work!

D and A's testimony:

We want to thank you from the bottom of our heart for treating both my husband and me during what possibly was our worst experience ever, faced with COVID-19. Both of us had more severe symptoms, which were only worsening. We were at the point where we could hardly sit up for even a couple of minutes—we had the worst body aches of our life, fever, and headache. We were isolated, treating our symptoms with OTC medications and drinking lots of liquids to stay hydrated. But with everything we were doing we had reached a place where, from one hour to the next, my husband reached a point where he was hardly responding.

That same day we had an appointment with Dr. Malos, and she prescribed hydroxychloroquine, zinc, and Z-pack. Within two to three days we felt much better, and we were back on our feet. The way we had felt, I did not believe that. Dr. Malos was right and truly was a lifesaving mediator for us in fighting COVID-19. After a couple of days of taking hydroxychloroquine, along with zinc and the Z-pack, we felt 90 percent better. We believe God sent Dr. Malos to provide us an escape from COVID-19 at the right time. May you continue to care, bless, and save people's lives with this treatment.

God bless you, D and A

S's testimony:

I am writing as a nurse and professor of nursing and a current caretaker for my parents, who within the last month had experienced signs and symptoms of COVID-19; my mother tested positive for the virus. They were immediately assessed and treated by Dr. Rodica Malos. Once the symptoms worsened, she started the treatment with hydroxychloroquine. Within twenty-four hours of being on the Zithromax and hydroxychloroquine regimen, both of my parents started feeling much better. Their fever broke, their cough got better, and they started to improve. I am certain that without this intervention, my parents would have needed to be hospitalized.

In addition to those two medications, they took vitamin D, vitamin C, and zinc, all of which were recommended by Dr. Malos. This treatment was imperative in the recovery of my parents, who are sixty-five and seventy years old. As a nurse and medical professional, I stand behind my testimony that this regimen was what saved my parents' lives and also kept them from going into the hospital. Please allow this treatment to continue to be prescribed for so many who are in need.

Pastor C's testimony

Dear Dr. Malos,

I wanted to take the time to express my appreciation for the help that you have given me and my wife, as well as to several other members from our community. As you know, on August 27 I contacted my doctor at KP, because I was not feeling well. Immediately, I was scheduled for a COVID-19 test and the result was positive. Very concerned at the news because of my history of sudden cardiac arrest, I contacted my doctor's office for treatment and advice. They basically told me to isolate and to wait for my symptoms to aggravate, and only then to call my doctor.

In the meantime, I was told to drink tea with honey and to take Tylenol or other over-the-counter cold medications. I could not believe what I was hearing! After all the warnings and all the stories from OHA (Oregon Health Authority) about people dying from this virus, I considered that advice very inadequate. For that reason, I called you for a second opinion. I was very fortunate to be able to speak to you on that same day and to receive treatment immediately, which included azithromycin, hydroxychloroquine, benzonatate, and zinc.

After two days of taking this treatment my fever was gone. In two more days, all my other symptoms had disappeared, with the exception of some headaches and a sore throat. In less than a week, my energy level was back, and I was healed. After fourteen days of isolation, I returned safely to the community and to my work. I want to thank you for being there for me and for all of your patients. I thank God for health professionals who care like you do.

Pastor C

Expressing Appreciation

During the outbreak of COVID-19 in our community, with the early interventions and patients recovering from mild and moderate symptoms, I heard many other similarly-powerful testimonies from patients. They reported their appreciation for early treatment and their full recovery, with many thanking God for His goodness in their lives. When they called, I could distinguish the calm in their tone of voice. Up to this day, I am receiving testimonies from patients whom I treated at home. They are thankful and grateful to God that they found someone who cares.

Even if my interventions only saved a single life, it was worth the risk of losing my license. It still baffles me the way those in authority reacted. Consider the discussions that could be explored:

- How early interventions that saved lives offer a way to extend the procedures and treatments to be implemented in every outpatient clinic
- Ways the practice of early interventions can prevent hospitalization and premature deaths in our state
- Development of a massive program for all health care providers

Instead, the state authorities searched for ways to intimidate me through three investigations, persecution, and revoking my license. This is sad, especially considering that delayed intervention often led to hospitalization—or worse. We dealt with many panicked patients whose COVID-19 symptoms got worse as a result of the "sicken-in-place" approach. When that happened and they had difficulty breathing, they sought help at our primary care clinic, even on Friday evenings after we had closed. Those who waited too long needed to go to the ER, but the damage to their lungs had already taken place.

They needed to be hospitalized for more aggressive and stronger treatment, because they did develop viral pneumonia and further complications. They needed a longer time to recover too. Their health condition and quality of life are not the same after the damage to their lungs from the debris and residuals from the inflammatory process in the alveoli that caused pneumonia.

Patients who developed pneumonia from COVID-19 infection broke my heart, knowing that they were the victims of the misguided approach that led to increased severity of the symptoms and fast deterioration, leading to lung damage and pneumonia, becoming hospital-dependent as a result. If they had had early access to HCQ, IVM, antibiotics, steroids, and other treatment—as recommended in the algorithm I presented earlier—they could have avoided hospitalization. And, further damage to their body, soul, and spirit.

Their health conditions and quality of life would be much different today.

Looking back on my experience in a short period of time with hundreds of patients treated at home early when their symptoms started, and who recovered completely, I am confident that early intervention works. We could have reduced hundreds of thousands of hospitalizations and deaths around the United States and other nations in the world. Add up the losses: economically, financially, emotionally, intellectually, mentally, and spiritually, and the toll is staggering.

Chapter 14

The New Variant: Love and Compassion

To learn that those in authority were not on the public's side during the pandemic shocked me. We should have been doing everything possible to save as many lives as we could, with all the knowledge, expertise, supplies, and medications available. Yet I observed a distinct lack of compassion for human life, whether that involved government authorities or those overseeing health care. My biggest concern was for my family, friends, and patients in our area. So many were in distress when virus-linked diseases struck them. This broke my heart, both for them and their suffering families. It was so disturbing that the medical establishment seemed not to care for those suffering from this legal pathogen. Words can't adequately explain the horror I felt.

The reassuring element in all this was knowing that God speaks—whether through His Word, the Holy Spirit, or other believers—in the bleakest of situations. Even though I have seen God move in countless ways through the years, I am still amazed by the multiple means by which He works. After hearing numerous testimonies from patients who recovered from COVID-19 through early interventions, I reflected back on what He did to even connect me with Good News Clinic in the first place. He guided me with His small voice to the right place to practice medicine during the pandemic, for the purpose of saving lives.

To understand the full picture, you need to know that my husband and I had taken a year-long sabbatical after working in our very demanding business for twenty-eight years. We had provided care to people with multiple chronic conditions. Many presented challenging behavior and needed memory care because of Alzheimer's disease or dementia. The relentless schedule (close to 24/7) proved physically and emotionally draining.

When we returned from our much-needed time of rest, I discovered that Portland Adventist Community Service Health Clinic (where I had volunteered for sixteen years as a general practitioner) had transitioned from medical care to a dental and eyecare clinic. As a result, I started to pray for God's guidance to direct me to a new clinic, where I could continue to volunteer my time helping vulnerable and needy people. A few months into this process, I sensed the Holy Spirit saying, "Dr. Sayson."

I was pleasantly surprised, because I had met him more than ten years earlier, when we wanted to learn a new program from his practice to adapt to our free clinic. I remembered that he prayed when we had a problem with the program on his computer, and the computer instantly sprang to life. That kind of bold prayer had an impact on my spiritual life. I vividly remembered that prayer for a decade. I knew he was a man of faith and prayer.

I paid attention to that small voice that resonated in my head; I knew God was speaking to me and that I had to listen and obey. As the prophet Isaiah assured us, "Your ears shall hear a word behind you, saying, 'This is the way, walk in it,' whenever you turn to the right hand or whenever you turn to the left" (Isa. 30:21). I contacted Dr. Sayson's clinic right away to discuss completing an application. Just a few weeks after proceeding with the paperwork and job orientation, the news about COVID-19 shocked everybody. Especially primary care providers, who were left without guidelines for early treatment to prevent hospitalization. Then, after lockdowns temporarily closed our clinic, we implemented telehealth.

Preventive Medicine

I was very happy to still be able to provide medical care through this method to help prevent unnecessary catastrophes in patients' lives. Any intervention was better than doing nothing to help suffering people, many who lived in terror. God had orchestrated His divine intervention to connect me with Dr. Sayson's clinic, so I could follow His guidance to help hundreds of people in terrible distress. Only God knew what was coming over the earth and our community before it started, so He prepared me ahead of time.

I am glad that I listened to the "still small voice" that guided my steps. It brought to mind the famous passage from Psalms: "The steps of a good man are ordered by the LORD, and He delights in his way. Though he fall, he shall not be utterly cast down; for the LORD upholds him with His hand. I have been young, and now am old; yet I have not seen the righteous forsaken, nor his descendants begging bread. He is ever merciful, and lends; and his descendants are blessed. Depart from evil, and do good; and dwell forevermore" (Ps. 37:23–27).

As the weeks passed and I tried to explain the wisdom of early interventions, skeptical experts would appear with "prudent" concerns, often asking, "Where is the evidence?" Trying to explain God's wisdom in human terms often doesn't make sense to rational thought processes. They can't grasp that "the LORD gives wisdom; from His mouth come knowledge and understanding" (Prov. 2:6).

Now, being led by the Spirit during the pandemic does not mean that I underestimated science or lowered our standards of care. I had always followed national guidelines and used the best scientific evidence in providing care to suffering patients in my business and the outpatient clinics where I practiced for decades. Our practice in medicine is always guided by science and the best scientific evidence. Our life is surrounded by science. God created science. God is above earthly science. He gives wisdom and spiritual intelligence to people on earth to develop science; that is, as much as He allows. He is sovereign and has the highest authority. He wanted us to look beyond earthly science when we were in a crisis—especially during a pandemic, when people were dying prematurely (and unnecessarily). And when we didn't have time to wait for randomized clinical trials that take a few years to develop. In those extreme situations when people were dying in front of our eyes, we had to depend on God, our Creator.

In primary care health clinics, providers faced dictates to disengage from caring for patients with COVID-19. I felt chills running down my spine again amid threats from health care authorities that we had to wait for randomized clinical trials to develop the best evidence. But the novel virus spread so fast it was killing millions around the world. I agree 100 percent with the authorities that we should obey science—I am a scientist by education and degree—but people were dying while we sat on our hands. To save lives I had to follow my God-given instincts, intelligence, and knowledge gained from three decades of experience. And, those experts who were willing to share their knowledge, experience, and expertise.

Alternative Approaches

Everyone felt the cruelty of the virus. We had no time to wait for randomized, controlled trials. Alternative approaches were urgently needed to save lives. We were left with common sense, instinct, knowledge, and experience of past qualitative studies and scientific evidence. Also, we knew of positive outcomes from experience in our practice. The authorities denied all of the above. It felt like reliving my experience in a communist country, where government propagandists told us we were not allowed to save souls by warning them that the wages of sin is death (see Romans 6:23). This at a time when vast numbers of people were living immoral lives and lying represented the societal norm.

Communist rulers told me if I talked to people about my hope in Jesus or about my values and beliefs based on Judeo-Christian principles that I would lose my job and be left with no resources and sentenced to death. Since communists didn't provide any social services, if you lost your job, you could easily starve to death. Once again during the pandemic, I had to live in a similar darkness and terror, with no solutions for sick patients. I felt the condemnation from other primary care practitioners who were denying treatment to patients with COVID-19, telling them to take OTC medications, use home remedies, and drink plenty of fluids. Based on common sense, that was the minimum one would do for mild symptoms. But when it came to COVID-19, we did not have science for those kinds of approaches.

As I mentioned earlier, the news media continued to suppress information that encouraged providers and patients about early interventions to save lives. After listening to news reports and reading articles containing so much negativism about President Trump's assertions about hydroxychloroquine, I decided to look for more evidence about this medication. In chapter 11, I mentioned a 2005 article in the *Virology Journal* about HCQ's strong antiviral effects on SARS-CoV infection of primate cells. In my new search, I found an article by a doctor describing how—also in 2005—the Centers for Disease Control's special pathogens division described three mechanisms by which chloroquine might work and have both a prophylactic and therapeutic role in coronavirus infections.

"More than 20 relevant studies have been published in journals indexed in PubMed between January 28 and April 20, 2020," wrote Jane M. Orient, MD. "AAPS (Association of American Physicians and Surgeons) concludes that: 'the safety of (hydroxychloroquine) is well documented. When the safe use of this drug is projected against its apparent effect of decreasing the progression of early cases to ventilator use, it is difficult to understand the reluctance of the authorities in charge of U.S. pandemic management to recommend its use in early COVID-19 cases."[43]

---

[43] Jane M. Orient, MD, "COVID-19: Where's the Evidence on COVID-19 Treatment?" Heartland Daily News, Heartland Institute, April 29, 2020, https://heartland.org/opinion/covid-19-wheres-the-evidence-on-covid-19-treatment/.

She added that observational results reported from China, France, South Korea, Algeria, and the US showed that of 2,333 patients treated with HCQ, 2,137 (91.6 percent) improved clinically. There were 63 deaths, with all but 11 documented in a single report from the Veterans Administration where patients were already severely ill, she wrote. Dr. Orient noted data near the end of April of that year showing US death rates were at least eight times higher than in countries permitting early and prophylactic use of HCQ. She added, "Opinion leaders should be demanding to know why this treatment option is not widely discussed or might even be forbidden."[44]

Extensive Evidence

Writing in the fall of 2020 in the Washington Examiner, Yale University professor Dr. Harvey Risch (now professor emeritus) noted that seven controlled, well-conducted clinical studies involving more than eleven thousand patients in seven nations all showed 50 percent higher reductions in hospitalization or death. He said not a single fatal cardiac arrhythmia attributable to the HCQ was reported and a new summary analysis of five randomized, controlled trials had also shown a statistically significant outpatient benefit, proving the case.

He charged that public criticism of President Trump by seven former FDA commissioners and the New England Journal of Medicine for "failing at every step" was in reality driven by craven politics and Big-Pharma-linked conflicts of interest. Dr. Risch said they were diverting attention from the FDA's "despicable" efforts to block access to effective and inexpensive generic medications, particularly hydroxychloroquine.

"Many or most of the 220,000 deaths in the United States to date could have been prevented by widespread HCQ use that the FDA blocked," Dr. Risch said. "It is the FDA that is responsible for these deaths, not the president. It is sheer corrupt hypocrisy, and completely

---

[44] Ibid.

shameful, for past FDA commissioners and for a New England Journal of Medicine editor with ties to the FDA to accuse the president of what the FDA itself has done. It is time to clean up this mess once and for all. The FDA must remove its black-box warning, approve the emergency use authorization for outpatient HCQ use, and let doctors get on with the work of saving lives."[45]

In chapter 5, I mentioned meeting Dr. Robert Malone, who happened to be the original inventor of the mRNA vaccine technology as a medical and graduate student in the late 1980s. In his book, Lies My Gov't Told Me, he wrote about the aforementioned 2005 paper in the Virology Journal by five CDC (US government) scientists and three Canadian government scientists, showing that chloroquine was an effective drug against SARS coronaviruses.

"The CDC paper is entitled 'Chloroquine is a potent inhibitor of SARS coronavirus infection and spread' and concludes with the following quote: 'Chloroquine has strong antiviral effects on SARS-CoV infection ... suggesting both prophylactic and therapeutic advantage,' Dr. Malone wrote. "A similar study was conducted in 2004 by a group of European scientists. In 2014, scientists working at the National Institute of Allergy and Infectious Diseases (NIAID), showed the same results. Not only did chloroquine work in vitro against the MERS coronavirus, but dozens of existing drugs, which could have been tested in patients as soon as the pandemic started, were also effective against SARS and MERS coronaviruses."[46]

The Case for Ivermectin

Before his death in 2022, Dr. Vladimir Zelenko saved thousands of lives with early interventions in his practice. He and two colleagues demonstrated that "the well-tolerated (five-day) triple therapy

[45] Harvey Risch, "FDA Obstruction: Patients die, while Trump gets the blame," Washington Examiner, October 19, 2020, https://www.washingtonexaminer.com/opinion/503349/fda-obstruction-patients-die-while-trump-gets-the-blame/.

[46] Robert Malone, MD, MS, Lies My Gov't Told Me: And the Better Future Coming, (Skyhorse Publishing, December 6, 2022), 70-71.

resulted in a significantly lower hospitalization rate and less fatalities with no reported cardiac side effects compared with relevant public reference data of untreated patients. The magnitude of the results can substantially elevate the relevance of early use, low dose hydroxychloroquine, especially in combination with zinc. This data can be used to inform ongoing pandemic response policies as well as future clinical trials.

"For outpatients with a median of only (four) days after onset of symptoms, COVID-19 represents a totally different disease and needs to be managed and treated differently. A simple to perform outpatient risk stratification, as shown here, allows rapid treatment decisions and treatment with the triple therapy of zinc, low dose HCQ, and azithromycin and may prevent a large number of hospitalizations and probably deaths during the SARS-CoV-2 pandemic. This might also help to avoid overwhelming of the health care systems."[47]

Earlier, I mentioned ivermectin in protocols used in early interventions by Dr. Zelenko and Dr. Peter McCullough. Research showed that ivermectin has anti-viral and anti-inflammatory properties, improving patients' symptoms from the COVID-19 virus. In an article published in the American Journal of Therapeutics, Dr. Pierre Kory and four other researchers noted that a meta-analysis based on eighteen randomized, controlled treatment trials of ivermectin on COVID-19 patients had discovered statistically significant reductions in mortality and time to clinical recovery and viral clearance. In addition, results from numerous controlled prophylaxis trials had reported significantly reduced risks of contracting the virus with the regular use of ivermectin.

"Finally, the many examples of ivermectin distribution campaigns leading to rapid population-wide decreases in morbidity and mortality indicate that an oral agent effective in all phases of

---

[47] Roland Derwand, Martin Scholz, and Vladimir Zelenko, "COVID-19 outpatients: early risk-stratified treatment with zinc plus low-dose hydroxychloroquine and azithromycin: a retrospective case study," International Journal of Antimicrobial Agents, Volume 56, Issue 6, December 2020, published online at Science Direct, https://www.sciencedirect.com/science/article/pii/S0924857920304258.

COVID-19 has been identified," they wrote. ... "More recently, trial results of ivermectin, a widely used antiparasitic medicine with known antiviral and anti-inflammatory properties, have been showing benefits in multiple important clinical and virologic outcomes, including mortality. Although growing numbers of the studies supporting this conclusion have passed through peer review, approximately half of the remaining trials data are from manuscripts uploaded to medical preprint servers, a now standard practice for both rapid dissemination and adoption of new therapeutics throughout the pandemic."[48]

Kory and the others also discovered large "natural experiments" had occurred when regional health ministries and governmental authorities in Peru, Brazil, and Paraguay initiated ivermectin distribution campaigns in hopes the drug would prove effective: "The tight, reproducible, temporally associated decreases in case counts and case fatality rates in each of those regions, compared to nearby regions without such campaigns, suggest that ivermectin may prove to be a global solution to the pandemic. This was further evidenced by the recent incorporation of ivermectin as a prophylaxis and treatment agent for COVID-19 in the national treatment guidelines of Belize, Macedonia, and the state of Uttar Pradesh in Northern India, populated by 210 million people."[49]

Searching for Solutions

Dr. Kory's experience in tirelessly providing care to patients with COVID-19 in intensive care units—and seeing many of the patients dying under his care due to complications—led him to the challenge of searching for data from different parts of the world. He wanted to access information about the effectiveness of ivermectin as a possible

---

[48] Pierre Kory, et. al., "Review of the Emerging Evidence Demonstrating the Efficacy of Ivermectin in the Prophylaxis and Treatment of COVID-19," American Journal of Therapeutics, April 22, 2021, published online at https://pmc.ncbi.nlm.nih.gov/articles/PMC8088823/.

[49] Ibid.

solution to stopping the pandemic. I heard one interview where he sounded emotionally drained and on the edge of tears as he told of begging the US Senate to review the data that he had obtained. He hoped to prove that ivermectin was an effective drug for COVID-19 symptoms, providing benefits to treat the disease and for prophylactic treatment.

My experience with using ivermectin came with a patient I will call Mrs. DF. She had experienced advanced symptoms from COVID-19, with her oxygen levels dropping below 88 percent at night. Extremely tired and weak, she was desperate for effective medical care. It was too late to start her on HCQ alone, but following Dr. Zelenko's protocol (mentioned in chapter 4) I added 12 milligrams of ivermectin, taken daily for three days. Mrs. DF's oxygen levels increased from 88 percent to 93 percent in less than twenty-four hours after the first dose, to 95 percent after the second dose, and to 97 percent after the third dose. It was like a miracle.

Mrs. DF recovered well and was so happy. She praised the Lord for His mighty intervention through available (and affordable) medications. She had been scared to death at the thought that she might need to go to the ER and be hospitalized for her severe symptoms. This is another example of the benefits from the protocols and algorithms developed by top doctors with lifetime experience. They used medications off-label to treat symptoms based on the pathophysiology of the diseases caused by COVID-19. My heart is full of thanks to God and those prominent physicians, general practitioners, and specialists who worked tirelessly to find solutions for symptoms from Covid. They were advocates for the most vulnerable populations suffering from this lethal pathogen.

Chapter 15

Searching for Justice

In the darkest time of the pandemic, God prepared the way so patients could escape the trials of COVID-19. Although they came like "a thief in the night" (2 Peter 2:10), God inspired doctors with expertise and experience in medicine to discover solutions for symptoms from the virus via early interventions and treatment. God inspired many doctors to develop protocols as preventive measures. I believe that to stop early interventions at home in favor of the do-nothing approach favored by the medical establishment represented an injustice for patients who were suffering with such severe symptoms. Many expressed their frustrations—and the fear that tormented them—over at-home treatment being denied by practitioners in primary care clinics, urgent care facilities, and emergency rooms.

Not only was withholding early intervention dangerous, it represented an injustice for patients in considerable physical and psychological distress. Especially those who later had to be hospitalized and died.

As people cried out to God for justice and truth in their desperation, the biblical passage that came to mind concerned Cain and Abel's story: "'If you do well, will you not be accepted? And if you do not do well, sin lies at the door. And its desire is for you, but you should rule over it.' Now Cain talked with Abel his brother; and it came to pass, when they were in the field, that Cain rose up against Abel his brother and killed him. Then the LORD said to Cain, 'Where is Abel your brother?' He said, 'I do not know. Am I my brother's keeper?' And He said, 'What have you done? The voice of your brother's blood cries out to Me from the ground. So now you are cursed from the earth, which has opened its mouth to receive your brother's blood from your hand. When you till the ground, it shall no longer yield its strength to you. A fugitive and a vagabond you shall be on the earth'" (Gen. 4:7–12).

Just as Cain killing Abel represented a serious injustice, so did allowing coronavirus patients to suffer needlessly and even die prematurely. In the health care field, we all have responsibilities to do well for our patients and treat their symptoms from any virus, let alone the deadly one that swept across the planet in 2020. In order to be accepted as God's servants, physicians and medical practitioners have an obligation to treat patients in physical and psychological distress. It is what we were trained to do.

Every Life Matters

My philosophy in life has always been that every patient's life matters. We must think in such terms at all times. Once I received a call from a Romanian immigrant, a Christian experiencing desperation over losing her husband. A once healthy, strong man, he had been weakened by COVID-19 infection. In the first week of mild and moderate symptoms, his primary care provider offered no early intervention treatment. As time passed, his symptoms grew worse, with his oxygen levels dropping to 90-92 percent (normal range is 98-99 percent). He went to the ER and was admitted to the hospital. Five days later they placed him on a ventilator. Two weeks after that he died, leaving behind a devastated family.

This is just one example of a very active, healthy, sixty-year-old male whose life could have been saved by early intervention. This is why it still pains me to think about the mainstream media, medical authorities, and leading academic experts suppressing the truth about the effectiveness of early treatment using repurposed prescriptions. I cried and grieved with that dear family, thinking, "Who are we in primary care to withhold early interventions from sick patients when they need it the most?"

As I have said previously, telling patients to wait at home until they were sick enough to go to the ER meant that in many cases damage to the vital organs had already been done by the inflammation and micro thrombosis caused by the aggressive virus. That severely diminished their chances of survival. Even if they lived, many were left with post-COVID-19 symptoms and Long Covid damage from the inflammatory phase and residuals from debris from the disease process.

The health care system failed to train doctors about the complex disease process from the lethal pathogen attacking the human body. We also failed to provide patients the education and insights necessary to understand the disease process and empower them to make well-informed decisions about their own care. Since COVID-19 variants will continue to be with us, we must provide care to every single patient with symptoms from COVID-19 with this truth in mind: every single patient's life matters, and truth and justice in medicine must be the focus of those in authority.

Preventive Measures

We were overwhelmed with sorrow during the pandemic, due to the lack of guidelines for primary care practitioners about intervening at the most crucial time—as a devastating virus started to kill millions worldwide. Instead, we were told to "do nothing." One day as I agonized over this troubling lack of concern for the public's welfare, the Lord brought to mind a passage from Nehemiah. Though at the time the people's hearts were full of sorrow, Nehemiah (the governor), Ezra (the priest), and the Levites told them the day was holy to the Lord and not to mourn or weep: "Go your way, eat the fat, drink the sweet, and send portions to those for whom nothing is prepared; for this day is holy to our LORD. Do not sorrow, for the joy of the LORD is your strength'" (Neh. 8:10).

As mentioned previously, I have always paid close attention to health promotion and disease prevention. These are important subjects and major keys to treating every illness that affects humans. During COVID-19, it was important to use common sense and to follow instructions for preventative measures. Among them were wearing a mask around sick people when social distancing was not possible, social distancing with people who were sick, washing one's hands frequently, disinfecting surfaces, avoiding big crowds when acuity was high, avoiding sick people, staying home if you are sick, and improving one's immune system with a healthy diet, regular exercise, and stress management.

These were all good practices to prevent contracting the virus. However, the uncertainty of how long all those practices will be prolonged affects our society directly and indirectly. It can often lead to anxiety and depression with long-term consequences. Dr. Harvey Risch (mentioned in the previous chapter) wrote in the spring of 2024 that in so many words the CDC had admitted that all the indignities of COVID-19 management—be it masks, social distancing, lockdowns, or closures— had failed.

"What the CDC recently reported ... however, is that by the end of 2023, cumulatively, at least 87 (percent) of Americans had anti-nucleocapsid antibodies to and thus had been infected with SARS-CoV-2," he wrote. "(This) in spite of the mammoth, protracted and booster-repeated vaccination campaign that led to about 90 (percent) of Americans taking the shots. My argument is that by making policies based on number of infections a higher priority than ones based on the more serious but less common consequences of both infections and policy damages, the proclaimed goal of the vaccine mandate to reduce spread failed in that 87 (percent) of Americans eventually became infected anyway."[50]

[50] Dr. Harvey Risch, "CDC Demonstrates Failure of Public Health Management of the COVID-19 Pandemic," Peter Navarro Substack, April 1, 2024, https://petenavarro.substack.com/p/cdc-demonstrates-failure-of-public?r=1a7xso&utm_campaign=post&utm_medium=web&triedRedirect=true.

He said it wasn't like we didn't know all this was going to fail, since as the events unfolded in early 2020 public health management of this respiratory virus was almost completely opposite to principles that had been established through an influenza period in 2006. The spread of a new virus with a reproduction number of about three and more than one million cases nationwide—with no potentially virus-sterilizing vaccine in sight for months—almost certainly made this infection endemic and universal, Risch wrote.

"In reality, neither vaccine immunity nor post-infection immunity were ever able fully to control the spread of the infection," he added. "On August 11, 2022, CDC stated, 'Receipt of a primary series alone, in the absence of being up to date with vaccination through receipt of all recommended booster doses, provides minimal protection against infection and transmission (3,6). Being up to date with vaccination provides a transient period of increased protection against infection and transmission after the most recent dose, although protection can wane over time.' Public health pandemic measures that 'wane over time' are very unlikely to be useful for control of infection spread, at least without very frequent and impractical revaccinations every few months."[51]

Isolated and Separated

On a more practical note, such steps as mask-wearing had a particularly inhibiting effect on social relationships, further dividing people into isolation and accentuating their fear. I rarely saw acknowledgement of the negative impacts (aside from the fact that I don't think they made much of a noticeable difference in preventing the spread of the virus). When someone wears a mask, others miss seeing their smile—and vice versa. Our mirror neurons in our brains have the role of helping us to smile when others are smiling at us.

---

[51] Ibid.

One scholar noted that groundbreaking research in the 1990s discovered that these neurons fire whether monkeys performed an activity themselves or observed others engaging in it. "In the decades since, studies suggest that humans also have mirror neurons, and they are fundamental to what it means to be human (Penagos-Corzo et al., 2022)," wrote Jeremy Sutton, PhD, who teaches psychology at the University of Liverpool in England. "Neuroscience shows that mirror neurons impact our ability to grasp new skills, acquire knowledge, and form deep emotional connections with those around us, even helping us understand why people do what they do (Cook et al., 2014)."[52]

It is fascinating how science reflects what we read in the truth of Scripture. As Paul wrote in his letter to the Romans: "Bless those who persecute you; bless and do not curse. Rejoice with those who rejoice, and weep with those who weep. Be of the same mind toward one another. Do not set your mind on high things, but associate with the humble" (Rom. 12:14–17).

Joy is one of the most powerful emotions that bring healing to our body, spirit, and soul. Joy is the antidote for sadness and depression. The reward mechanism in our brain is activated when we are full of joy and dopamine is released. That enhances our motivation for the activities of daily living and everyday life. Serotonin and endorphins, oxytocin, and other neurochemicals are released in the body to restore our health and to keep us healthy. Smiling is extremely important in our daily life, to prevent the anxiety and depression that affect our body, soul, and spirit in a negative way. Joy brings health and strength to our being. The Bible teaches us about the importance of being happy and rejoicing always.

After five years of the pandemic situation worldwide, there were still many things to learn about the transmission of the COVID-19 virus and the severity of the illnesses it causes. That is the dilemma for all experts, scientists, and professional people working in the

---

[52] Jeremy Sutton, PhD, "Mirror Neurons and the Neuroscience of Empathy," Positive Psychology, September 7, 2023, https://positivepsychology.com/mirror-neurons/.

health care field. Due to a lack of specific, scientific evidence, people are more anxious than ever. Without clear solutions, their concerns are nearly as strong as when lockdowns erupted overnight. We must emphasize some aspects of the transmission of this virus:

- The signs and symptoms that develop after COVID-19 exposure and infection
- The signs and symptoms of an emergency
- How to protect ourselves to prevent coronavirus infection
- The importance of our immune system in fighting this unpredictable virus, and
- Preventing comorbidities and complications caused by COVID-19 in those with comorbidities

It is interesting to note that many people thought that once pandemic restrictions eased that the issues surrounding COVID-19 had ended. With all the research, investigation, and scientific studies yet to be completed, they are only beginning.

Chapter 16

Spirit of Wisdom

"He who gets wisdom loves his own soul;
he who keeps understanding will find good" (Prov. 19:8).

Throughout the pandemic, the plethora of unknowns and uncertainties sparked an endless series of questions from patients. It is easy to understand such concern; as of June 1 of 2024, nearly 1.2 million persons in the US had died from COVID-19.[53] That is why we can have the "peace of God, which surpasses all understanding" (James 4:7) when we seek wisdom from above in hard times. Here are short responses to the most common questions people asked about the COVID-19 virus and the diseases it caused. (The CDC displays all of these recommendations online, easily accessible at https://www.cdc.gov/covid/index.htmlge).

1. **What do we need to know about COVID-19? How is it transmitted?**

We learned from the CDC that the virus is transmitted from person to person at a distance of less than six feet. It is transmitted through respiratory particles produced by an infected person when they are coughing, sneezing, or talking. These particles get into our mouth and nose and are inhaled into our lungs from the particles spread by infected persons in the atmosphere around us.

---

[53] "About COVID-19," Centers for Disease Control, https://www.cdc.gov/covid/about/index.html, accessed December 20, 2024.

2. How fast is this virus transmitted?

COVID-19 is transmitted faster and more easily than influenza, and more slowly than measles, which is very contagious.

3. What are the signs and symptoms?

* Fever.
* Dry cough, although this can be productive if irritation causes a person to produce mucus that helps expel phlegm.
* Sore throat.
* Shortness of breath. Many patients will report, "I cannot breathe" while others state, "I cannot get enough air in my lungs" or, "The air is staying at the entrance of my lungs," or, "I have pressure in my chest" or, "There is burning inside my chest when I breathe" or, "I feel burning inside of my upper back."
* Hypoxia, which is when the oxygen level drops from ninety-seven to eighty-nine; in many cases this takes place seven to eight days into the progression of the disease. Those people need to be on alert to go to the hospital right away, because the oxygenation is compromised in vital organs, tissues, and cells. This can create multi-organ failure and death. People may try to use a nebulizer and an oxygen machine at home. But even with those interventions, if the oxygen level drops below 92 percent, people must go to the hospital for further evaluation and intervention.
* Chest pain or pressure.
* Cyanosis, which is a bluish discoloration of the lips or skin.
* Chills and sweats.
* Headaches.
* Pink eye.
* Muscle and joint pain. Many patients have reported to me that "it is like someone is pulling my flesh away from me," which causes excruciating pain.

* Syncope, or a temporary loss of consciousness (fainting). When this occurs, people get up to perform the activities of daily life and instead fall on the floor.
* Extreme fatigue and tiredness where the sufferer is unable to get up to use the bathroom.
* Dizziness.
* Anorexia.
* Loss of smell and taste loss.
* Nausea, vomiting, or diarrhea.

Silent Symptoms

All of these symptoms are real; a majority of patients who sought interventions and treatment at our clinic experienced them. Because COVID-19 symptoms manifest in so many ways, every person's condition is different. They can present at a mild, moderate, or severe level, meaning there is no universal "blueprint."

Early in the pandemic, a study by researchers at the University College London found only a small fraction of those infected developed severe symptoms, which usually occurred in people who were at higher risk because of comorbidities. The Coronavirus Infection Survey tested 36,000 people living in England, Northern Ireland, and Wales from April to June of 2020. It revealed that 86 percent of those tested positive for COVID-19 did not have virus symptoms, such as cough, fever, and loss of taste or smell.

"The study findings, collected by the Office for National Statistics, the U.K. statistics body, highlight the role of asymptomatic patients in the spread of the virus," wrote Angela Laguipo in a report for the Medical and Life Sciences website. She said the authors of the study—published in the peer-reviewed, open access journal Clinical Epidemiology—wrote, "To reduce transmission of SARS-CoV-2, it is important to identify those who are infectious. However, little is known about what proportion of infectious people are asymptomatic and potential 'silent' transmitters." [54]

While pinning down the causes and symptoms of coronavirus is extremely challenging, the truth we can stand on is knowing that our body is created in a complex way. This innate strength can enable us fight trillions of virus cells and stay strong so we don't even exhibit symptoms. The Psalmist wrote about God's amazing work in our body 3,500 years ago: "Thank you for making me so wonderfully complex! Your workmanship is marvelous—how well I know it. You watched me as I was being formed in utter seclusion, as I was woven together in the dark of the womb. You saw me before I was born. Every day of my life was recorded in your book. Every moment was laid out before a single day had passed" (Ps. 139:14–16 NLT).

Emergency Signs

During his bout with COVID-19, Mr. J experienced great distress—especially from not knowing when to call 911 or go to the ER after staying home and waiting for the symptoms to get worse. When he called me to ask, worry consumed his every waking thought. Many other patients were in similar distress. Either they or people they knew had gone to the ER, only to be told they were not sick enough to be hospitalized and sent home. This created considerable confusion and psychological distress.

The following list contains the CDC's recommendations for those with possible warning signs of COVID-19. If someone is showing any of these signs, seek emergency medical care immediately:

- Trouble breathing
- Persistent pain or pressure in the chest
- New confusion
- Inability to awaken or stay awake

---

[54] Angela Betsaida B. Laguipo, BSN, "86 percent of the UK's COVID-19 patients have no symptoms," News: Medical and Life Sciences, October 9, 2020, https://www.news-medical.net/news/20201009/86-percent-of-the-UKs-COVID-19-patients-have-no-symptoms.aspx.

- Bluish lips or face*[55]

Many patients develop difficulty breathing after COVID-19 affects their lungs, yet do not recognize that. When I discussed their symptoms with patients who called to report that they had tested positive, I asked if they had a cough. Often they responded no, but after a few more questions, I would hear them coughing intermittently; they were not aware that they had a dry cough. Others had a "wet sound" or a "tired larynx" when they talked, which indicated they had symptoms, yet were not aware of them. Many developed foggy brain from the inflammatory process of the Covid viral infection.

I strongly advised patients to check and monitor their oxygen levels daily—even two or three times a day—using a pulse oximeter (a small device available at a pharmacy, medical supply store, or ordered online). When oxygen levels drop below 96 percent, it is an indication that the virus has multiplied, provoking the immune system to cause a more intense inflammatory process in the lungs. The damage in the lungs starts from the bottom, at the alveolar level where the exchange of oxygen and carbon dioxide happens, and the oxygenation is impaired by the damaged alveoli by the virus's multiplication in the lung cells. That is the time to be hypervigilant and watch for more declines in oxygen levels and signs of hypoxia, such as cyanosis and bluish lips and face. Call your primary care doctor or go directly to the ER.

Treatment Levels

The majority of patients with compulsive cough episodes, dyspnea, and oxygen levels decreasing to 92 percent showing signs of inflammation in the lungs can be treated with steroids at home. This can include such items as prednisone or dexamethasone, inhalers,

[55] *This list does not cover all possible symptoms. Please call your medical provider for any other symptoms that are severe or concerning. Call 911 or call ahead to a local emergency facility. Notify the operator that you are seeking care for someone who has or may have COVID-19. See more information at https://www.cdc.gov/covid/signs-symptoms/index.html, accessed December 23, 2024.

budesonide via nebulizers, or oxygen supplementation, if they have no life-threatening conditions. If the patient's condition declines to where they are unable to get up to use the bathroom, develop severe chest pain, or have increased fever of more than 101 degrees Fahrenheit—even with maximum treatment of Tylenol or NSAIDs (nonsteroidal anti-inflammatory drugs), such as ibuprofen or Advil—they need to go to the hospital immediately. Patients who are ignorant of aggravating symptoms and refuse to go to the hospital are at a high risk of death.

Some patients experienced syncope (fainting). One patient reported that she went to the bathroom and fainted when using the toilet; another went to shave and fainted in the bathroom, with a family member finding them on the floor. One patient's blood pressure dropped to a below normal reading of 78/46 and he got so weak he could not stand up. His wife found him on the bathroom floor, where he had fallen while shaving. Other patients reported that they were so sick that they were unable to stand up and move around to perform the activities of daily living, or to cook for themselves.

With several of the latter patients, when I asked them to go to the emergency room, they refused. This despite my urging that it was absolutely necessary for their survival to get treated at the hospital. Some patients expressed concern that if they went to the hospital their condition would further deteriorate, and they would end up on a ventilator and die. In those situations, I had to step in and start treatment right away to save their lives, which only happened because of God's grace.

Call Your Doctor

"But the wisdom that is from above is first pure, then peaceable, gentle, willing to yield, full of mercy and good fruits, without partiality and without hypocrisy" (James 3:17).

Just as James advised, we must use wisdom during a health crisis. If you continue to experience any of the COVID-19 symptoms I listed earlier, even after early intervention or prophylactic treatment, you must go to the hospital. People must know that each case is different—because each person is uniquely created, with unique DNA containing instructions for life, and a unique immune system response when activated by the virus. Each person's genetic makeup is different and responds differently to a virus infection.

Regardless, you need to be aware that many patients can become so sick they experience life-threatening symptoms. Signs and symptoms can manifest anywhere from two to fourteen days after exposure to the virus. It will then follow its course, according to the condition of your health and immunity levels that can fight off the virus. Pay attention to the signs and symptoms of COVID-19. I generally gave patients the following instructions (although more can be added as appropriate):

1. Patient instructed to follow CDC recommendations for isolation to prevent spreading of the virus.

2. Patient instructed to go to ER if:

* Temperature is over 101 Fahrenheit (even if taking OTC meds for fever)
* Respiration rate is more than thirty breaths per minute (even if taking bronchodilators via inhalers or nebulizers)
* Oxygen level is lower than 90 percent (even with oxygen supplementation)
* Have bluish discoloration of lips or skin
* Experiencing chest pain, chest pressure, shortness of breath, increased fatigue, increased dizziness, fainting, and other severe symptoms

Hold medication if heart rate is lower than sixty beats/minute or if experiencing irregular heartbeats (contact medical provider immediately), and take 325 mg. aspirin daily to prevent blood clots during COVID-19 symptoms. It is very important to talk to your doctor about all your signs and symptoms during this period, and afterwards to detect any residuals from the diseases caused by COVID-19. Do not ignore any symptoms, as they may give you signals about damage done in your body by the virus even after the illness has passed.

Biblical Prevention

Long ago, the wisest man who ever lived (Solomon) told us there is nothing new in human history: "What has been will be again, what has been done will be done again; there is nothing new under the sun" (Eccl. 1:9 NIV). Likewise, from ancient times we have learned that we must avoid people with contagious diseases and that they must be isolated. This was the case with Moses and Aaron in Old Testament times: "The LORD said to Moses and Aaron, 'When anyone has a swelling or a rash or a shiny spot on their skin that may be a defiling skin disease, they must be brought to Aaron the priest or to one of his sons who is a priest. The priest is to examine the sore on the skin, and if the hair in the sore has turned white and the sore appears to be more than skin deep, it is a defiling skin disease. When the priest examines that person, he shall pronounce them ceremonially unclean. If the shiny spot on the skin is white but does not appear to be more than skin deep and the hair in it has not turned white, the priest is to isolate the affected person for seven days. On the seventh day the priest is to examine them, and if he sees that the sore is unchanged and has not spread in the skin, he is to isolate them for another seven days'" (Lev. 13:1-5 NIV).

It is quite interesting that our usual treatment regimen for early intervention for COVID-19 virus infections and symptoms was five to seven days; if the patient continued to experience symptoms, we repeated the treatment for five to seven more days. Patients isolated themselves during this time as being contagious. The portion of Scripture I just quoted was written about 3,500 years ago, giving the precise time of seven to fourteen days of isolation during sickness with contagious disease.

As for protecting yourself, in the previous chapter I mentioned such steps as avoiding contact with sick people, avoiding group gatherings during a virus outbreak, and maintaining your distance from those who are sick, or staying home yourself if you are sick.

A word of caution about masks: they are not good for children under two years of age, people with respiratory problems, or those unable to remove a mask without assistance. A mask plays a role in protecting others around you if you are infected with COVID-19 or other contagious diseases and have symptoms. But it does not replace the distancing method when you are sick. You do not need to wear your mask if you are alone in a private space, car, office, home, or walking alone on the street.

As for good sickness prevention methods, whether you have the Covid virus or just a head cold, follow these steps:

* Always cover your mouth and nose with a napkin when you cough or sneeze, or cough or sneeze into your elbow.
* Throw all tissues used to cover cough or sneezing into the garbage.
* After using the restroom or other situations where you soil your hands, immediately wash them with soap and water for twenty seconds.
* For disinfecting surfaces, use solutions that contain at least 60 percent alcohol if soap and water are not available. Disinfect daily all frequently used surfaces, such as: tables, doorknobs, light switches, cooking surfaces, desks, telephones, and keyboards. Also, toilets, handles, faucets, and sinks.
* Clean dirty surfaces first with detergents or soap and water, then disinfect.
* Use household disinfectants from stores. Keeping surfaces clean is a wise practice for good hygiene at home and in public, even when it is not pandemic time.

* Verify at all times all the recommendations from the National Centers for Disease Control and Prevention.[56]

Despite these useful guidelines, the saddest part is that the CDC did not mention a single word about early interventions to save lives. And nobody from the medical profession—whether doctors, nurses, pharmacists, scientists, experienced medical experts, or the medical establishments—raised the question: "Why?"

[56] "Symptoms of COVID-19," Centers for Disease Control, https://www.cdc.gov/covid/signs-symptoms/index.html , accessed October 10, 2020.

Chapter 17

Strength for the Fight

"Now there are varieties of gifts, but the same Spirit; and there are varieties of service, but the same Lord; and there are varieties of activities, but it is the same God who empowers them all in everyone"
(1 Cor. 12:4–6 ESV).

I like the way the above biblical passage brings out the truth about fighting COVID-19 and other viruses: there are a variety of tools that can strengthen your immune system in order to fight off deadly infections. At this time there is no clear evidence nor pharmacological strategies to prevent and treat the diseases caused by COVID-19 with 100 percent success. Nobody knows exactly when the alarming situation with this virus will end. Because of this reality, the most important thing is to explore strategies to improve your immune system to fight this unpredictable and invisible enemy.

There are prophylactic measures you can take to prevent diseases from striking. To prevent severe complications caused by COVID-19 and other viruses or bacteria, it is extremely important to reduce obesity and metabolic syndrome, such as hypertension, diabetes, or dyslipidemia. The latter is a condition characterized by high levels of fats in the blood, which can stem from genetics, medication conditions, or lifestyle factors, i.e., poor diet, lack of exercise, or smoking.

In my first book, Find Your Peace, I wrote in detail about preventing metabolic syndrome through lifestyle changes and stress management to deal with fear, anxiety, and depression. Checking blood pressure, blood sugar, and cholesterol levels is extremely important to managing these negative influences through a healthy diet, exercise, and medication when necessary. It is important to check vitamin levels and to prevent vitamin deficiencies through fresh fruits and vegetables and probiotics. A balanced diet with healthy nutrients and proper hydration are extremely necessary. It is wise to seek medical advice about micronutrient supplementation and caloric intake, according to your condition and any special health conditions.

Strengthening Immunity

To strengthen the immune system I recommend:

- Multiple vitamins play a huge role in strengthening the immune system for vulnerable persons with vitamin deficiencies. This includes persons with restrictions in their diet, such as vegetarians, infants, children, adolescents, pregnant or breastfeeding women, and the elderly.
- Many people have deficiencies of micronutrients, such as vitamin D, due to a lack of exposure to the sun. It is important to use vitamin D 2000 IU daily; also, your primary care physician should check vitamin D levels through blood tests.

In his book, *Fight Back: Beat the Coronavirus*, Dr. Chauncey Crandall—a renowned cardiologist and director of Florida's Palm Beach Clinic—recommends various supplements to optimize the immune system. "To fight back against COVID-19, you need every weapon you can lay your hands on," he writes, "and this means taking supplements, which can give you an important nutritional edge. These recommendations can strengthen your immune system to help fight off COVID-19 ... These are the essential supplements you need to keep your immune system strong. They are also useful if you feel the symptoms of a cold, the flu, or even what you suspect might be COVID-19 coming on. It's also always important to take a multivitamin every day to cover any deficiencies you might have (but) of which you are unaware."[57]

- Daily use of vitamin C (1,000 mg), vitamin D (5,000 IU; your primary care doctor should check vitamin D levels, vitamin A (25,000 IU), zinc (40 mg), selenium (200 mcg), magnesium (200 to 400 mg), quercetin (500 mg), and garlic (9,000 to 18,000 mg).[58]
- Fresh vegetables and fruits are rich in antioxidants that strengthen our immune system. It is important to stay hydrated with fluids in order to remain physically active to prevent clot formation. Use frequent rest periods and preserve energy when fatigued. To improve the immune system to be able to fight coronavirus, daily intake of fresh vegetables and fruits high in anti-oxidants (with the power to neutralize free radicals that cause "oxidative stress") is recommended. Examples are tomatoes, red peppers, garlic, onions, broccoli, kale, red potatoes, spinach, green beans, and colorful fruits. Dark chocolate with no sugar is also helpful, as are products containing probiotics—plain yogurt, buttermilk, pickles, sauerkraut, kombucha, tempeh, and kefir.

Comorbidity Prevention

The elderly; others with medical conditions such as heart disease, diabetes, and lung diseases; or those with compromised immune systems are at higher risk to develop serious complications from diseases caused by COVID-19. As Dr. Crandall wrote in his book about coronavirus, one study noted that patients who were hospitalized because of the virus had certain preexisting conditions, including obesity, heart disease, and diabetes: "Such conditions are often associated with the 'metabolic syndrome' that afflicts one-third

[57] Dr. Chauncey Crandall and Charlotte Libov, Fight Back: Beat the Coronavirus (Humanix Books, 2020), 72-73.

[58] Ibid.

of adult Americans. People with metabolic syndrome have two or more of the following conditions: obesity, high blood pressure, diabetes, high triglycerides, and low HDL cholesterol, the 'good' cholesterol."[59]

Knowing your numbers is another key to good health. By that, I mean various blood sugar, cholesterol, and other readings that are good indicators of health. It is important to maintain the following:

- An average blood pressure of 120/80 mmHg for adults (acceptable range is from 90/60 to 140/90).
- Blood sugar levels at 70-99 mg/dl before breakfast.
- Total cholesterol less than 200 mg/dl. LDL (bad cholesterol) less than 100 mg/dl and HDL (good cholesterol) more than 40 mg/dl.
- Triglycerides less than 150 mg/dl, etc. Only through lab work ordered by a primary care doctor can people know the values of their cholesterol, glucose, enzymes, electrolytes, minerals, and vitamin levels. To maintain a normal blood pressure, normal blood sugar level, and normal cholesterol to prevent heart disease and diabetes, it is important to follow a healthy diet daily. This means:
- Reducing the consumption of salt with all meals to prevent hypertension. (During a COVID-19 situation, be aware that you must check electrolyte levels and blood pressure more frequently, because the virus may reduce sodium levels. This can cause hyponatremia and hypotension, leading to confusion, lethargy, and extreme fatigue. If hyponatremia and hypotension happens you must consume salty food; in this particular case, if you get coronavirus symptoms.)
- Reduce red meat and animal products.
- Reduce greasy foods, such as fats, sauces, cheese, creams, butter, cookies, and cakes.

---

[59] Ibid.

- Increase the consumption of vegetables to three to five portions per day.
- Increase fruit consumption to two to four portions per day (for diabetics, reduce that to one to two portions per day and less sweet fruits)
- Avoid greasy and oily foods.
- Reduce carbohydrates, such as potatoes, bread, pasta, and rice.
- Use oils sparingly: fish oil, avocado, seeds, nuts, and olive oil.
- Follow a healthy diet with fresh vegetables and fruits.
- Reduce consumption of animal proteins, and increase protein consumption from legumes and vegetables. Some examples are spinach, peas, soybeans, sprouting broccoli, avocado, beans, garden asparagus, lentils, cauliflower, Brussels sprouts, potatoes, maize, cabbage, and artichokes.
- Fruits are rich in vitamins, but you must also consider the amount of sugar they contain.

Obesity is a comorbidity that causes many complications in patients with COVID-19, and can lead to death. To reduce body weight and obesity, a person must reduce portions of all foods in order to reduce the amount of calories ingested (except fresh vegetables, which are low in calories). The consumption of a low-calorie diet will help a person to reduce weight, which will help to reduce blood pressure and blood sugar levels and lead to better control of hypertension and diabetes.

Intermittent Fasting

The benefits of intermittent fasting are well documented in medical literature; this practice helps our physical and spiritual health. The Bible also gives many examples of fasting and guidance for engaging in intermittent fasting. I often think of biblical examples of those who fasted for spiritual battles and received the secondary benefit of improved physical health. One example is the "Daniel fast," which means to eat only fruits and vegetables for twenty-one days.

The book of Daniel outlines the plan: "In those days I, Daniel, was mourning three full weeks. I ate no pleasant food, no meat or wine came into my mouth, nor did I anoint myself at all, till three whole weeks were fulfilled. ... So Daniel said to the steward whom the chief of the eunuchs had set over Daniel, Hananiah, Mishael, and Azariah, 'Please test your servants for ten days, and let them give us vegetables to eat and water to drink. ... And at the end of ten days their features appeared better and fatter in flesh than all the young men who ate the portion of the king's delicacies. Thus the steward took away their portion of delicacies and the wine that they were to drink, and gave them vegetables" (Daniel 1:2–3, 11–12, 15–16).

You can read the entire book of Daniel to get a fuller perspective on the benefits of fasting. However, before undertaking any kind of fast, talk to your doctor about your condition; you may want to consult with a specialist to see if fasting will create any concerns with your health. The sooner you check on this the better, since you will know what kind of intermittent fasting you can engage in to improve your immune system, besides getting stronger spiritually.

Remember too that hydration is vital during a time of fighting COVID-19 and other viruses. Total fluids should amount to two thousand milliliters a day, the equivalent of eight eight-ounce glasses of liquids. For proper hydration I often recommend Pedialyte, which contains electrolytes—minerals essential to health—and glucose that keep your body hydrated longer than plain water.

Whatever you do, for any health decision follow sound medical advice from certified medical providers, primary care practitioners, doctors, physicians, nurse practitioners, or general practitioners. They can offer you recommendations regarding supplements, vitamins, and nutritional supplements. A doctor who knows you personally can offer tailored guidelines regarding exercise, medication, treatment, diagnosis, and medical interventions and procedures. No matter what your status, though, the following are wise steps to take for good health:

- Exercise and physical activity every day—at least ten thousand steps or sixty to ninety minutes a day
- Avoid a sedentary life with little exercise
- Avoid smoking
- Avoid alcohol intake
- Use stress management procedures
- Follow medical advice from your doctor for treatment for diseases that aggravate complications produced by COVID-19 and for dealing with post COVID-19 symptoms

Post COVID-19

After several months of the pandemic, we had no information in the primary care environment to guide our practice for post-acute COVID-19 symptoms and what to expect from patients who had recovered from COVID-19. As time passed, though, we gained some insights. We started to hear from many patients (who had started interventions and treatments in the second week of symptoms) that some symptoms persisted three to four weeks after recovery—or even longer.

A year after the virus reached our shores, a health industry publication reported that 80 percent of COVID-19 patients had lingering symptoms or signs fourteen or more days after acute infection, based on a systematic review and meta-analysis. Sonia Villapol, PhD, of Houston Research Institute and her colleagues reported that more than fifty symptoms tied to SARS-CoV-2 infection persisted. Most common were fatigue (58 percent), headache (44 percent), attention disorder (27 percent), and hair loss (25 percent).

"Preventive measures, rehabilitation techniques, and clinical management strategies designed to address prevalent long-term effects of COVID-19 are urgently needed," she told MedPage Today. "To date, there's no established diagnosis for the slow, persistent condition that people with lasting effects of COVID-19 experience;

terms like '(Long) COVID,' 'long haulers,' and 'post-acute COVID-19' have been used, Villapol and colleagues noted. In their review, they referred to lingering symptoms and signs as 'long-term effects of COVID-19.'"[60]

Indeed, some patients who experienced symptoms after their infection were asking me why some symptoms were still present for weeks or months after the COVID-19 season had ended. Among these were dry or wet cough, perspiration, fatigue, tiredness after completing small tasks, shortness of breath upon exertion, and needing to rest often between tasks. In many cases the patients reported intermittent chest tightness even two months after the virus was gone.

As the pandemic unfolded, we were learning that many organs besides the lungs were affected by COVID-19; there are many ways the infection can affect someone's health. While most persons with COVID-19 recover and return to normal health, some patients can have symptoms that can last for weeks or even months after recovering from acute illness. Even those who are not hospitalized and only have mild illness can experience persistent or late-onset symptoms. Multi-year studies have been initiated to further investigate. The Centers for Disease Control continues to work to identify how common these symptoms are, who is most likely to get them, and whether these symptoms will eventually resolve.

The most commonly reported long term symptoms include:

- Fatigue
- Shortness of breath
- Cough
- Joint pain
- Chest pain

[60] Judy George, "80% of COVID-19 Patients May Have Lingering Symptoms, Signs," MedPage Today, January 30, 2021, https://www.medpagetoday.com/infectiousdisease/covid19/90966.

Other reported long-term symptoms include:

- Difficulty with thinking and concentration (sometimes referred to as "brain fog")
- Depression
- Muscle pain
- Headaches
- Intermittent fever
- Fast-beating or pounding heart (also known as heart palpitations)

More serious long-term complications appear to have been reported, and affect different organ systems in the body. These include:

- Cardiovascular: inflammation of the heart muscle
- Respiratory: lung function abnormalities
- Renal: acute kidney injury
- Dermatologic: rash, hair loss
- Neurological: smell and taste problems, sleep issues, difficulty with concentration, memory problems
- Psychiatric: depression, anxiety, changes in mood

Unwelcome Houseguest

The longer the pandemic drags on, the more obvious it becomes that for some patients, COVID-19 is like the unwelcome houseguest who won't pack up and leave, said one industry report.

"'Anecdotally, there's no question that there are a considerable number of individuals who have a post viral syndrome that really, in many respects, can incapacitate them for weeks and weeks following so-called recovery and clearing of the virus,' Anthony Fauci, MD, director of the National Institute of Allergy and Infectious Diseases, said in July (2020) during a COVID-19 webinar organized by the International AIDS Society."[61]

The report—written by Rita Rubin for the JAMA Network (which encompasses the Journal of the American Medical Association) also noted that "overall, approximately 10 (percent) of people who've had COVID-19 experience prolonged symptoms, a UK team estimated in a recently published Practice Pointer on post-acute COVID-19 management. And yet, the authors wrote, primary care physicians have little evidence to guide their care."[62]

While adults with severe illness can spend weeks in intensive care and experience long-lasting symptoms, that's not unique to patients with COVID-19, Rubin added. She wrote that what was unusual about the "long haulers" is how many initially had mild to moderate symptoms that didn't require lengthy hospitalization, let alone intensive care. She quoted Jessica Dine, MD—a pulmonary specialist at the University of Pennsylvania Perelman School of Medicine—as saying most of the patients she saw who are suffering from post–COVID-19 syndrome were not hospitalized.

"Why some previously healthy, often young, adults still haven't recovered from the disease has stymied physicians," Rubin wrote. "'We in the medical field are very accustomed to taking care of respiratory syncytial virus and other pneumoviruses in young adults,' Wesley Self, MD, MPH, an emergency medicine physician at Vanderbilt University Medical Center, said in an interview. With those infections, 'people feel pretty sick for (two) to (three) days, and then they feel markedly better.' But COVID-19 is another matter..."[63]

As we learned from the patients we treated, post COVID-19 symptoms are all too real. They need close monitoring and frequent follow-up visits to provide reassurance, encouragement, and sometimes more treatment, assessment, and evaluation. The latter may

---

[61] Rita Rubin, MA, "As Their Numbers Grow, COVID-19 'Long Haulers' Stump Experts, JAMA Network, September 23, 2020, https://jamanetwork.com/journals/jama/fullarticle/2771111.

[62] Ibid.

[63] Ibid.

span a variety of specialists, such as a cardiologist, pulmonologist, neurologist, nephrologist, endocrinologist, and others. That such a wide-ranging team can be needed for some situations demonstrates the formidable nature of the fierce foe that has caused such widespread destruction across the planet.

Chapter 18

COVID-19 Turmoil

We live in a world where many see lying as a virtue, when in reality it is deceptive and dangerous. Lying is immoral and unethical when practiced in society, but even more damaging when it comes to the medical field. During the pandemic, health and government authorities lied to general practitioners and others about early treatments and about vaccines. Not only did this make many question the claim the vaccine was "safe and effective," this went against what those of us with nursing and medical degrees learned in school: to be trustworthy. This was especially true when caring for patients. I always posed the question: "If you cannot trust a doctor or a nurse, whom can you trust?"

When the pandemic began, people anxiously awaited for the antidote: a promised vaccine to stop the pandemic. They clung to the hope this vaccine could stop the lethal pathogen destroying so many lives. Yet, when authorities began mandating the vaccine, I heard numerous concerns about mRNA vaccines; they ranged from one extreme to the other. The most-asked questions at that time:

- What is it made of; what does it contain?
- Are there enough studies done regarding long-term consequences?
- Is this an experimental vaccine?
- Why is there no informed consent?
- Are these synthetic vaccines? Are they effective?
- Why are so many young people dying suddenly when they perform tasks as athletes, musicians, or artists?

- Why are cancer incidents increasing so much since mass vaccinations?

Supposedly, synthetic COVID-19 mRNA vaccines use a novel approach by which mRNA is delivered into our cells to provide the genetic instructions for our own cells to temporarily make a specific viral protein that triggers an immune response. Scientists answered the question about the vaccine's ingredients, presenting a simple breakdown of the COVID-19 vaccine as stated in the following article:

"The Pfizer-BioNTech COVID-19 vaccine is made of the following ingredients: mRNA—also known as messenger ribonucleic acid, mRNA is the only active ingredient in the vaccine. The mRNA molecules contain the genetic material that provides instructions for our body on how to make a viral protein that triggers an immune response within our bodies. The immune response is what causes our bodies to make the antibodies needed to protect us from getting infected if exposed to the coronavirus.

"There are rumors that mRNA vaccines will alter our DNA because the RNA molecule can convert information stored in DNA into proteins. Scientists sustain that that the mRNA vaccines never enter the nucleus of the cell, where our DNA is stored. After injection, the mRNA from the vaccine is released into the cytoplasm of the cells. Once the viral protein is made and gets on the surface of the cell, mRNA is broken down and the body permanently gets rid of it, therefore making it impossible to change our DNA."[64]

Questions Remain

That was the ideal plan to develop the antidote for the lethal pathogen that circulated in different variants and affected millions of people around the world. Even if that was the truth about the synthetic

---

[64] Mai Abdel Haleem Abusalah, et. al., "Nucleic Acid-Based COVID-19 Therapy Targeting Cytokine Storms: Strategies to Quell the Storm," Journal of Personalized Medicine, March 3, 2022, https://pmc.ncbi.nlm.nih.gov/articles/PMC8948998/.

vaccines, questions remain about the duration of immunity created by the anti-COVID-19 vaccine.

This was recognized early on by Pfizer executive Phil Dormitzer. He commented during a December 2020 interview with MedPage Today: "There'll be many more questions about what is the duration of immunity. Do we start to see cases that're breaking through a long time out? Now, if we were to completely suppress circulation of this virus, well, there'll be no virus circulating to make people sick, but we don't know whether that's the case or not. It is possible. There will still be virus circulating in a significant degree in two years. Or that may not be the case, but regardless, we do want to see how long immunity does last, to the degree that the natural circulation of the virus allows us to do that."[65]

During the entire period of the pandemic, I felt quite frustrated that nobody seemed to be talking about the natural immunity of people who already had a Covid infection and recovered from their symptoms. In their previously mentioned (in chapter 2) book, Overcoming the COVID Darkness, Drs. Tyson and Fareed noted how "an Israeli study showed that natural immunity is at least thirteen times more powerful than vaccination at preventing infection."[66]

I arrived at the conclusion that when a deadly virus is circulating and infecting people worldwide while causing millions of deaths, we cannot wait for what I see as a questionable vaccine. We must use early treatments as an alternative, during and after the pandemic. This is similar to the way we approach other diseases caused by different viruses. Or, other causes to save people's lives.

In my opinion, the fact that authorities banned early treatment during the pandemic gives evidence of a criminal hand at work. People were forced to take what was an experimental vaccine against their

---

[65] Serena Marshall and Lara Salahi, "What Do We Really Know About Pfizer's New COVID Vax?", MedPage Today, Dec. 16, 2020, https://www.medpagetoday.com/podcasts/trackthevax/90243?xid=fb_o&trw=no&fbclid=IwY2xjawHfyg1leHRuA2FlbQI xMAABHRswNvS2hGwzN28KTUWpaGJ4-N738TCR_A6QHu0YDF8-Iq8CQYtAp1EO0A_aem_MM1R4fJC9XUxP9eybhXVsA.

[66] Overcoming the COVID Darkness, 80.

will. Those who refused the mandate were often forced to leave their jobs and states where they had built a career. They had to had to pack up and dislocate their family, with their children leaving behind friends and relationships built over a long period of time.

I was especially concerned that health authorities pushed the vaccines so hard but mentioned nothing about natural immunity and early treatment. Or, at least to consider other alternatives to prevent premature death until a truly safe, efficient, well-studied vaccine becomes available. Especially when some people could not take the vaccine, which was creating more spike proteins and having an enhanced effect that could overwhelm the immune system. This could produce more symptoms from the massive inflammatory process in the body, destroying vital organs. Many experts had the same concerns.

Yet vaccinations are continuing, even as increasing numbers of studies show that Long Covid and synthetic vaccines have serious consequences, as mentioned in the Vaccine Adverse Event Reporting System (VAERS). Though reportedly rare, among the adverse effects reported to VAERS are anaphylaxis, blood clots, myocarditis, pericarditis, hearing changes, and tinnitus.[67]

Inhumane Treatment

In addition, mandating an experimental vaccine without proper studies of long-term effects was inhumane. Jane Orient, the executive director of the Association of American Physicians and Surgeons (whom I quoted in chapter 14), has stated that government vaccine mandates are "a serious intrusion into individual liberty, autonomy and parental decisions."[68]

While she has often been labeled an anti-vaccine zealot and quickly dismissed by critics, I have an all-too-real story that backs up

[67] For more information, see "Review of adverse events associated with COVID-19 vaccines, highlighting their frequencies and reported cases" at https://pmc.ncbi.nlm.nih.gov/articles/PMC10507236/.

[68] Kenya Evelyn, "Anti-vaccine doctor to testify at Senate committee hearing on Covid mandates," The Guardian, December 7, 2020, https://www.theguardian.com/world/2020/dec/07/anti-vaccine-doctor-testify-coronavirus-senate-hearing-jane-orient.

Orient's contention. It is the sad saga of Dr. CCD, who had a devastating experience with the vaccine mandate during the pandemic. Her story breaks my heart. An incredible doctor in the urgent care field for twenty years, she is also a close friend. She wrote to me to relate her sad story, which I wanted to include in this book. I want to let readers know how much compassionate physicians who cared for sick people endured during this sad chapter of American history. Her story follows.

"A Big Dream"

"Once upon a time, when I was child I had a dream ... a big dream: that I am a doctor, a very good one and I help many people. People around me are all healthy and happy and able to help each other and live a plentiful life. Time passed and passed. Hard study, dedication, and discipline were needed and all made possible through the help of God, my Father, who inspired me through His love letters, who encouraged me and transformed deserts into a beautiful path for me.

One day I was holding the big diploma of a doctorate in medicine in my hands! I promised Him at that moment that I will not forget about the dream that I had as a child ... the dream that started me on this path. And I kept my promise. I worked diligently with a smile on my face, happy to fulfill my mission: to help people get better and to dissolve sickness around me. But one day, a dark heavy force with very long wavelengths and surges of widespread destruction crashed ashore onto our land: the Covid tsunami!

People were scared. Doctors and staff got scared. Covid infection was viewed like leprosy or even worse. At that time, my site was assigned to become the front-line place for patients with Covid and other diseases/signs/symptoms or suspected Covid. I had staff personnel and colleagues who left. Friends and family advised me to quit, to treasure my family and my children and flee to a safe place. But I stayed put, knowing I was there in that time and place for a reason.

I did this with scarce supplies, like one mask per day to see forty to fifty patients per shift. A few months into this battle I got sick. Not only did I contract Covid, so did my father. He was ripped apart by sickness. When I lost him, I felt that my root cracked deep. Daddy was a great support to me and prayed constantly for me, my patients, and my mission field. Now he was gone while I was left so very sick—emotionally and physically. I got weak, suffered from a foggy brain and migraine headache, and struggled to walk.

I could not get relief with antimigraine medication and found little help. We had very little Covid education about complications. But this was not the end of the hardship. Soon into this, I received a note about the Covid vaccine mandate. I asked for an exception: to be allowed to postpone the vaccine until I felt better and healthier. But I was told there were no exceptions. The director told me that without the vaccine I could no longer work and would be fired.

However, he agreed to grant my resignation so I would not be in such an undesirable position of being fired. So, I signed my resignation letter after working twenty years in the same workplace. Now, I felt *the ground under my feet shaking*! Sick with no remedies and no help for me, no job, no health insurance, no money, and three children in high school to take care of, and my husband off work too. What was coming next with this *disaster train on wheels*? No job without vaccines, in pain and with no medicine. I wondered if I would get to the point of being homeless and left with no house and no food. Several clouds of negative possibilities swirled into my sore mind and crying soul.

But what hurt me the most was *my dream shattered into pieces.* I couldn't help people anymore. I burst into tears of helplessness and despair until my knees hit the ground ... where I found God right there for me, and His care, compassion, and promises for me. Promises of only good plans! And I remembered again where I started: actually, I am here for Him. So, He helped me. This time, he wove the miracle (using His people) into my path to help me and guide me. Only a few months later I had a new job, a new home, and a new place to serve Him. Oh, He helped me. Because He can. And because *He loves to help me.*

What a tragedy for this super-qualified doctor, who to me is a hero for saving lives in an urgent care setting. Yet she faced persecution for being reluctant to take a mandated vaccine while sick with Covid and post-Covid symptoms. And while she was suffering from migraine headaches, knowing that you cannot take a vaccine with the same side effects.

The Wrong Focus

I was puzzled when, in such an urgent situation, we focused so much attention on an experimental vaccine that was not well-researched and forced people to take it, regardless of their condition. There were many people with reasonable objections (health or special circumstances, not just religious reasons) to taking the vaccine or the boosters that followed. Yet no one would consider using early interventions to save lives. I have to wonder how much of the resistance lie in political—namely, hatred of President Trump or conservative figures who recommended early intervention—rather than scientific reasons.

This all caused me to meditate on another situation when a wave of influenza struck our memory care facility several years ago. We had an outbreak of influenza A, starting with a pair of confirmed cases. In order to prevent the spread of influenza to the entire facility with thirty residents, we administered the flu vaccine to every person to immunize all residents prophylactically. But even with the vaccines people were still getting very sick. We administered the treatment for influenza prophylactically to everybody in spite of the vaccine, in order to avoid residents developing pneumonia and die. Despite our timely interventions, some elderly residents still passed away in a short time from pneumonia—being frail, old, and suffering from numerous disabilities for years. Other patients survived because they received treatment prophylactically even though they had taken the vaccine for influenza.

From this very simple example we can learn that we need to be more aggressive in treating people early at home if they get sick from the Covid virus, even if they can get a well-studied vaccine with high effectiveness in the future. We must be prepared in primary care to intervene early when people start to get symptoms from the virus or even prophylactically if the risk to get infected by virus is high, even with vaccination—especially since new mutations to the virus take place every year.

When obligated to take one of the COVID-19 vaccines, many patients expressed fear to me, both of the unknown about the content of the vaccines and mode of action behind them. We were instructed about the Covid vaccine that contains mRNA (enveloped in lipid nanoparticles in a vaccine that is delivered via injection) with genetic instructions for our own cells to produce temporary, specific viral proteins, to trigger our immune systems to produce antibodies to fight the COVID-19 virus when we are exposed. We were told that the Pfizer vaccine does not contain tissues from aborted babies, and does not contain the active or inactive COVID-19 virus. The mRNA does not get into the nucleus of the cells where our DNA resides. It does not affect our DNA. The mRNA disintegrates in about one week and disappears after we develop the antibodies necessary to protect our bodies from the virus.[69]

That was what we knew at that time about the vaccines for COVID-19. I was skeptical about the mRNA vaccine because of the need for more research. The results were controversial too, especially for a vaccine authorized for emergency situations only. And, without finishing all phases during the research period of its effectiveness and side effects for a longer time, even though nanotechnology "have been used in numerous clinical trials for anticancer, anti-inflammatory, antibiotic, antifungal, and anesthetic drug delivery, as well as for the

---

69 "COVID-19 Vaccine Basics," Centers for Disease Control, https://www.cdc.goFv/covid/vaccines/how-they-work.html, accessed March 24, 2021.

delivery of gene therapies."[70] But more research was needed after all those clinical trials.

Developing Antibodies

We were told that the reason to get two separate doses is because that would allow time for our body to develop antibodies after the first dose; then the second dose would give a boost to increase the level of antibodies. What we did not know is how much immunity we would get, and for how long. People became confused due to the controversial information, lack of transparency in disclosing side effects, information about possible adverse reactions, a lack of data about safety, and other factors.

People conducted their own research about vaccines and made their own decisions. We cannot be ignorant of information that is available for early intervention, prophylactic treatment, and/or the status of vaccines and their risks and benefits. We must have an understanding of why we take the medications or the vaccines we are advised to take, understand their effectiveness, and know about their possible side effects and adverse reactions.

Consent is extremely important when it comes to taking chemical substances into our body. Those who refused consent often faced the same persecution as Dr. CCD—in fact, thousands. Their rights were absolutely ignored. Such action flies in the face of all Americans' rights. As Dr. Simone Gold commented in her book, I Do Not Consent: "We are blessed to live in an extraordinary country that has guaranteed our human freedom by law. While fighting to maintain this freedom, every one of us must enjoy our freedom. When you enjoy your freedom of speech, freedom of religion, freedom of assembly, you remind yourself and others why we fight."[71]

---

[70] "Understanding the nanotechnology in COVID-19 vaccines," BioTech, https://biotech-spain.com/en/articles/understanding-the-nanotechnology-in-covid-19-vaccines/, accessed March 24, 2021.

[71] Simone Gold, MD, JD, I Do Not Consent: My Fight Against Medical Cancel Culture (Bombardier Books, 2021), 83.

Dr. Gold also encouraged professional practitioners to put patients first in their practice and to not be afraid. She wrote that Americans need not feel afraid, but empowered: "Their physicians should not be prevented from upholding their Hippocratic Oath and healing their patients. Instead, they must be permitted to practices sound and safe medicine. Patients and their doctors must be able to discuss the options for optimal care and treatment and the patient-physician relationship must take precedent."[72]

Patients must make well-informed decisions based on the truth. Throughout the Bible, God let people make decisions for life on earth, including accepting all the consequences for their choices. However, He continually encourages His people to choose life: "I call heaven and earth as witnesses today against you, that I have set before you life and death, blessing and cursing; therefore choose life, that both you and your descendants may live" (Deut. 30:19, emphasis added).

That is telling us how to choose life: we must know God's living Word. It contains a plethora of instructions on how to live and how to come closer to God. Knowing the Word of God is the key. Ignoring God's instructions in the Bible that teach us how to live a Christian life built on Judeo-Christian principles, values, and believes brings bad consequences. Sin has negative side effects and adverse reactions that lead to spiritual death.

We are complex beings with body, soul, and spirit, with a conscious mind. God designed those features in human beings while giving us the power of discernment and ability to make decisions for our lives on this earth. No matter what form they take, mandates represent dictatorship, the same kind I experienced under a communist regime—a horrifying form of government that leads to destruction. Those who fight for truth and freedom are often persecuted, when it is the dictatorial rulers who should face opposition.

---

[72] Ibid. 135.

Chapter 19

Unsafe Mandate

No sooner had I received the "safe and effective" COVID-19 vaccine than I started experiencing strange side effects. It began with tingling in my hands and feet and around my mouth, mimicking neurological signs and symptoms of neuropathy. I also felt sharp pains shooting in my head, mild dizziness, a mild cough, and slight nausea. Though I had considerable nervousness about taking the vaccine—and now my misgivings appeared quite valid—I had no choice but to take it because of the mandates issued for front-line medical professionals and others caring for patients. Because I felt compelled to provide care for suffering people during the pandemic, I had to comply.

As always, I had trusted the health care agencies that guided our care and medical practice. Yet there is no doubt in my mind that we were lied to during this time about the safety and effectiveness of this so-called promising vaccine. Knowing the studies for the vaccine were not finished, it really upset me when the mandates forced chemicals on people before an appropriate scientific basis had been established.

What's more, I knew there was something sinister about the mandates, as well as corresponding restrictions on early treatment. I knew we had been lied to by those in authority, the very people whom I had trusted during three decades of working in the health care field. Standing in line and watching people going through the hospital doors quietly like sheep to the slaughter, I prayed the verse from the Bible for no harm to come to them: "They shall take up serpents; and if they drink any deadly thing, it shall not hurt them; they shall lay hands on the sick, and they shall recover" (Mark 16:18 KJV, emphasis added).

Now, in my case, I knew that all medications and vaccines have side effects. And, as a general practitioner and a prescriber, I knew how to treat those symptoms. So I took prophylactic medications, such as hydroxychloroquine, dexamethasone, and Allegra, and the vaccine's side effects went away in a few days. I was able to cope with the symptoms because I knew what was going on in my body. But, I thought, "How scary for non-medical people when they experience these kinds of symptoms."

The health authorities offered no patient education whatsoever about the mRNA vaccine. The medical establishment and the news media did not utter a single word about treating side effects, just as they did not offer a single word about early treatment for those suffering from COVID-19 symptoms. The side effects of the vaccines were almost the same as the side effects of coronavirus, but nobody in top academic settings or mass media discussed such topics. All I heard was propaganda from the media and persecution of those who did the right thing to save people's lives.

For example, after he received the vaccine, my husband experienced such sharp chest pains that he thought he was having a heart attack. And he had been a CPR instructor for about two decades, teaching people signs and symptoms of a heart attack, and how to save lives! Given our respective experiences, we both felt quite displeased with the lies told about vaccines and mandates for people who had to go through this sinister process.

Contracting the Virus

The lie about the vaccine's effectiveness upset us even more when we both contracted Covid. Our entire family was working in the health care field, caring for sick and suffering people. Since we all faced mandates to take the vaccine, imagine our irritation when outbreaks struck us even though we had all received it. And when we got Covid, our primary doctors refused us treatment even though we were suffering from severe symptoms. We had to resort to seeking treatment via telemedicine with the same protocol that saved millions of lives around the world.

As Dr. Steven Hatfill, a specialist physician, virologist, and public health consultant with a broad range of experience in infectious disease control, disaster preparedness, and toxicology, noted in the spring of 2024, the mRNA vaccine program should have been halted in February of 2021: "By then early-use (hydroxychloroquine) and (ivermectin) had demonstrated an overwhelming safe effectiveness at reducing COVID-19 mortality with no adverse cardiac events. This supported a return to safe, early, drug treatments that would have controlled pandemic progression as it had in (fifty-one) other countries.

"Instead, the Biden Administration coerced and unconstitutionally mandated mRNA 'vaccination' with tragic results. When it became obvious the 'vaccines' were not reliably preventing infection, the CDC's mantra changed to one where mRNA 'vaccination' would 'prevent serious disease progression.' Yet there was no data to support this statement."[73]

Dr. Hatfill also noted that the worst thing is that by mid-2021 the FDA expanded its authorization for mRNA vaccines to include twelve-to-fifteen-year-olds and then lowered that to kindergartners. By June of 2022, he said it had been extended to infants and children between the ages of six months and four years, even though these age groups have almost zero mortality risk from COVID-19.

"Scientists have no idea what is happening with the injected infants and young children, except that basically it is 'safer to become infected with COVID-19 than to take the mRNA "vaccines,"' he wrote. "Where is the accountability for the false vaccine narrative? Irrespective of who holds the presidency, the COVID-19 debacle was

---

[73] Dr. Steven Hatfill, "The Politics of Pandemic Blame," Peter Navarro Substack, May 1, 2024, https://peternavarro.substack.com/p/the-politics-of-pandemic-blame?utm_source=share&utm_medium=android&r=15jluv&triedRedirect=true. See also "COVID-19 early treatment: real-time analysis of 4,082 studies" at https://c19early.org/.

caused by a handful of senior federal health bureaucrats who ignored the science and their oaths, in favor of the pharmaceutical manufacturers."[74]

Persecution Is Real

Prominent physicians, doctors, practitioners, scientists, and experts who stood up for the truth were harshly criticized and the targets of character assassination by the news media. Following is just one example of how media spread misinformation and disinformation about these professional people, even though they were saving thousands of lives with safe and effective medications. These "super heroes" stood for the truth and advocated for people's lives as they fought for freedom in medicine. Yet the media lied about them to incite more persecution, damage their reputation, and humiliate them in front of the world.

"I was defamed by the media, censored by social media companies, terminated by my employers, and viciously attacked," Dr. Simone Gold wrote in her book, I Do Not Consent. "(All) for advocating for the right of physicians to do what they always had done in America: prescribe what they believe is best for their patients. If it can happen to me, it can happen to anyone." [75]

A prime example is the sneering profile of America's Frontline Doctors (AFLDS) carried on Wikipedia, the well-known online encyclopedia. The site dubbed AFLDS a "right-wing political organization" and said it promoted falsehoods about the COVID-19 pandemic and vaccines (history will judge who promoted falsehoods). Although many of these doctors, including me, had used hydroxy-chloroquine, Zithromax, and zinc, Wikipedia called it a "cocktail" that could be used to cure COVID-19, which is not what any of us claimed. We simply said these off-label medications could help treat early

---

[74] Ibid.

[75] I Do Not Consent, 43-44.

symptoms instead of letting patients grow sicker and sicker, with some winding up in ICU or even dying.

"One of the speakers, Stella Immanuel, said that she herself had treated and cured 350 COVID-19 patients using the aforementioned cocktail, and referred to doctors refusing to use hydroxychloroquine as being like the 'good Germans who allow the Nazis to kill the Jews,'" they wrote. "They also accused 'fake pharma companies' of sponsoring studies that found hydroxychloroquine to be ineffective against COVID-19. The event was live streamed by Breitbart News, and video of the event was shared on social media platforms, such as Facebook groups dedicated to anti-vaccination and conspiracy movements, and on Twitter—where Donald Trump (who had also promoted the drugs) and his son Donald Trump Jr. both shared versions of the video.

"Citing policies against COVID-19 misinformation, Facebook, Twitter, and YouTube began to delete posts of the video. It was estimated that posts of the video on Facebook had reached over 14 million views before the takedown. Twitter restricted the account of Trump Jr. for 12 hours after he uploaded a version of the video to his account. When asked about the video, Trump referred to the group as being 'very respected doctors,' and referred to Immanuel as 'spectacular.' When asked why he trusted Immanuel despite her history of promoting conspiracies (such as alien DNA being used as part of medical treatments), Trump replied, 'I thought she was very impressive, in the sense that, from where she came—I don't know what country she comes from—but she said that she's had tremendous success with hundreds of different patients.' Following the event, Gold said that she had been fired from her position as an emergency room physician at two hospitals."[76]

[76] "America's Frontline Doctors," Wikipedia, https://en.wikipedia.org/wiki/America%27s_Frontline_Doctors, accessed April 23, 2024.

Misinformation or Censorship?

Due to the Frontline Doctors' courage to stand up for the truth and fighting for freedom and because of their willingness to share their expertise, knowledge, and experience, millions are alive today. We were treated with early interventions that prevented hospitalization and saved our lives from premature death from a deadly virus. Many of those who did not have access to early treatment died prematurely, with millions of families still grieving their loss. All because of the media's suppression and mislabeling America's superheroes who saved countless lives as spreading "misinformation."

The irony is they were sharing from their knowledge, expertise, and experience in saving countless lives across the world from dying unnecessarily. I must confess that I am alive today because of Frontline Doctors' heroic actions. So are members of my family and many of my patients. It is clear that around the world health authorities suppressed early interventions and helped disinform patients. Patients who were suffering symptoms that caused premature death or multiple diseases, with long-term complications. Add to that the psychological distress that helped create a mental health crisis. It was all unnecessary.

After analyzing data and reports, Dr. Robert Malone wrote that virtually anyone who had read his essays and books, or listened to his many podcasts, is aware of the profound failures, medical mismanagement, notable ethical breaches, and deep corruption that characterize the medical system and public health response to the COVID crisis.

"We are also aware that the various branches of the US medical system, pharmaceutical-industrial complex and the US Government /HHS system has deployed a wide range of propaganda, censorship, and PsyWar tools and technologies," he said. "(This blocked) both citizens and medical care providers from communicating about these failures and from proposing alternative solutions." [77]

This scandal has largely gone unnoticed and underreported. However, over time I believe the historical record will bring more of the truth to light and help lift the veil from millions of people's eyes. At least, I hope that is what happens.

---

[77] "US Healthcare during COVID - Lowest Performance, Highest Cost."

Chapter 20

Treatment for the Soul

As with every physical disease and health condition, when we are in emotional distress (besides prevention) early intervention is the key. As health practitioners, we have learned from anxiety, depression, and suicide that the treatment for the soul is as crucial as treatment for the body. If we address only the body, treatment is incomplete.

When patients with symptoms of the COVID-19 virus called me, by the tone of their voice I could sense their distress and agony. They were overwhelmed with emotion from fear, to the point of crying during the call. The agony of many patients with their physical pain, emotional distress, and suffering touched my heart.

The "virus of sin" is also an invisible enemy for the soul and spirit, one that has infected the entire world since creation. As with physical symptoms from infection, we must use the spiritual prescription written by the apostle James: "Confess your trespasses to one another, and pray for one another, that you may be healed. The effective, fervent prayer of a righteous man avails much" (James 5:16).

While the world was awash in turmoil because of the COVID-19 virus, many ignored the virus of sin, which has eternal consequences. The antidote is faith in the blood of the Lamb that came to rescue the world from eternal death. Nearly every patient expressed concerns and sadness due to their symptoms from the unpredictable virus, to the point of panicking as they expressed anxiety over the fear of disease and death. As a Christian, I knew that medical treatment would not adequately address such problems; those symptoms created emotional discomfort. In my spirit I felt their deep pain, and immediately said fervent prayers for a touch from heaven in their body, soul, and spirit.

You see, prayer is medicine, which can remove the burden of fear. Each time I prayed with a patient, I recognized the lifting of this burden when I said, "Amen." I could hear in each person's voice gratitude for this treatment for the soul, one they needed as much as the prescribed medications. I thought to myself that there must be something more, beyond science, to be able to help those in psychological distress from these scary symptoms and diseases caused by the COVID-19 virus. It put so much fear in people's minds, affecting their emotions and their quality of life. COVID-19 is a disease that steals joy from people of all ages. Prayer is needed, not only to practice our faith, but to eliminate fear and psychological distress.

Scientists have demonstrated that prayer and meditation produce significant reductions in blood pressure and heart rate, synchronize breathing and circulation, improve melatonin and serotonin levels, improve the immune system to fight infections from viruses and bacteria, reduce stress, promote good moods, and reduce anxiety and pain in degenerative diseases.[78]

When we pray with our patients (who agree to allow us to pray for them), our love touches their emotions in a way that medications alone cannot. They realize that we do not trust only the medications we prescribe. We trust the One who gives insights to the physicians and scientists who develop those medications; His love extends to us all. When we pray, the patients feel that we extend our care beyond science to care not only for the body, but also for the soul and spirit. We show the love of Jesus in providing holistic care with unconditional love. We know the truth: doctors treat diseases but Jesus heals them.

---

[78] Dr. Scott Hannen, Stop the Pain: The Six to Fix, (Trilogy Publishing Group, 2019), 270.

Give Unconditional Love

In his position, the only approach to working with someone else is to give them unconditional love, says William A. Petri Jr., a professor of medicine in the division of infectious diseases and international health at the University of Virginia. Petri, who holds an MD and PhD, is also vice chair of the department of medicine.

"That's what was given to me by Christ, dying on the cross for me," says Dr. Petri of the need to treat patients with this kind of acceptance. "If you're giving someone unconditional love, it is so freeing. If this person says something that irritates you, that slight doesn't matter because this is all about, 'What can I contribute (to) this person?'"[79]

That was exactly what I was doing: providing care and prayer with unconditional love. When patients with signs and symptoms of the COVID-19 virus called, after discussing their condition in detail and my plan for treatment, I would also ask if they would let me pray for them. There are two reasons why I offered prayer: 1) my heart was broken for their physical and emotional suffering, and 2) I felt a sense of desperation for them because of the virus's unknown mechanism of actions and unpredictable progression. It could destroy cells, tissues, systems, and organs, leading to long-term consequences for some patients. For others, it could lead to multiple trips to the ER, hospitalization, complications, ventilators, and in some cases death. At this point, medical providers were hopeless and helpless.

Many times, during these prayers, I would hear patients weeping as they poured out their heart to God. One patient said between sobs, "That is what I needed the most: prayer. I am healed now." Her emotional healing had a huge impact on her physical recovery from her symptoms. No longer hindered by fear, she started to function normally. Weakness and lethargy from anxiety and depression vanished, making her able to concentrate and perform

[79] "Prayer from the Front Lines of Coronavirus Research (Dr. William Petri)," Christian Civics Podcast, March 14, 2020, available at https://www.imdb.com/title/tt29752053/.

activities of daily living. Fear cripples people and even paralyzes them. What a huge difference a prayer makes when you are desperate!

Prayer in the name of Jesus Christ was an essential part of my early interventions. I heard many testimonies from patients of how prayer helped them. One patient (V), who had prolonged symptoms of extreme fatigue and weakness, told me, "The healing process started when we prayed on the phone." Three other patients (A, G, and L) were in desperation after their fever had not subsided for more than a week, even though they were taking maximum doses of Tylenol. All three said, "The fever stopped after we prayed." When I followed up, the patients stated that they were doing well—the medications had helped in two to three days, but "prayer helped right away." Another patient reported that his heart rate had normalized the same day we prayed for that. In his book, Stop the Pain, Dr. Scott Hannen noted that it is quite possible to find fifteen minutes to pause and pray to reduce the stress that causes inflammation and damage to the organs in our body.[80]

Improved Immunity

We know very well now that COVID-19 causes anywhere from mild to severe inflammation to our body's organs. This is due to a weakened immune system, which overreacts and does not work properly. It is well documented in medical literature that prayer helps our immune system to get stronger through the healthy neurochemicals released in our body when we focus on the things of God— our Creator, the source of our peace and health. Increased fear suppresses immunity through the emotions of anxiety, sadness, and depression, but prayer enhances immunity's effectiveness through thanksgiving and joy.

Prayer is closely aligned with healing; healing depends on prayer. When I pray with patients, I tell them that I always pray the medication I prescribe will do the job that it is supposed to do, but

---

[80] Stop the Pain, 271.

healing comes from God, our Healer. Doctors treat and God heals. The Bible says that when the Israelites were sick with many diseases, God sent His Word to heal them. As David wrote in the Psalms: "He sent His word and healed them, and delivered them from their destructions. Oh, that men would give thanks to the LORD for His goodness, and for His wonderful works to the children of men! Let them sacrifice the sacrifices of thanksgiving, and declare His works with rejoicing" (Ps. 107:20–22).

God's Word is His prescription for health and has the power to heal all our physical and spiritual diseases. I obeyed the Holy Spirit and prayed fervently throughout the day for every single patient I knew who was sick during the pandemic. I decided to trust God in caring for our patients. I remember how I had clung to my faith during the communist regime in Romania, when government officials' tyrannical attitudes intimidated and humiliated me nearly every day. How sad to encounter similar attitudes in a country on Judeo-Christian ethics, values, and beliefs. Holistic care is the key to addressing every patient's needs—physically, mentally, spiritually, and socially. Emotions are real factors contributing to a person's well-being.

I heard patients giving testimonies after prayers when I followed up daily on their conditions—how their symptoms improved and their joy was restored. Staying in touch with each patient via daily texts or calls provided them considerable relief from the fear of disease caused by the deadly virus. I observed firsthand how patients responded to me checking on them with daily follow-up, prayer, and Bible verses, in addition to the physical treatment and prescriptions. This all gave them hope in God's promises for divine health and complete healing.

Reading my daily texts or hearing my voice on the phone arouse hope in their minds and hearts, which changed their emotional states. I could hear the calmness in their voice and expressions of hope. I made it a habit to text them a verse from the Bible—the living Word of God with power to heal diseases—or encouraging, positive words with

God's promises, to increase their faith and to decrease fear. Faith is the antidote for fear.

God's Mystery

Prayer is the most powerful tool in all circumstances. I used to tell people that prayer is God's mystery, for every human being to enter into His spiritual realm and connect with His supernatural power for supernatural intervention. He gave us the command to pray, not to understand everything we are praying about. Our Creator wants us to communicate with Him. From ancient times we learned that the invisible God intervened right away when the priests and the people took actions to obey His Word. As it says in Numbers: "Then Aaron took it as Moses commanded, and ran into the midst of the assembly; and already the plague had begun among the people. So he put in the incense and made atonement for the people. And he stood between the dead and the living; so the plague was stopped" (Num. 16:47–48). The incense means the prayers; this is outlined in Revelation: "Now when he had taken the scroll, the four living creatures and the twenty-four elders fell down before the Lamb, each having a harp, and golden bowls full of incense, *which are the prayers of the saints*" (Rev. 5:8, emphasis added).

Prayer in Christ's name is the most crucial element of treatment. One time at a medical conference I heard Dr. Crandall, the cardiologist I mentioned in chapter 17 (and director of the world's largest heart transplant program), say that we must give people "the best of Christ and the best of medicine." By faith in prayer, we can ask God to intervene on our behalf even during situations like the pandemic. I am convinced that God intervened in the US during this fear-inducing time; early in the pandemic *The New York Times* reported that "the White House models they displayed showed that more than 2.2 million people could have died in the United States if nothing were done." I believe that millions of people around the world prayed, and

God spared the population of the USA and the earth from even worse destruction.[81]

Perhaps one of the finest words on prayer comes from English preacher C. H. Spurgeon. Although he lived during the nineteenth century, he retains influence in many Christian circles today. In his book, *Prayer*, he commented: "We want to draw near to You now through Jesus Christ the Mediator, and we want to be bold to speak to You as a man speaks with his friend. Have You not said by Your Spirit, 'Let us therefore come boldly unto the throne of grace' (Hebrews 4:16)?"[82]

Those words are as true today as when Spurgeon wrote them more than a century ago. When we seek healing, peace, and comfort from coronavirus and other diseases that may arise in the years to come, let us draw boldly before God's throne of grace. When we know His peace which—in the words of Philippians 4:7—"surpasses all understanding," we will be able to withstand the dread, threats, and pressures that have caused many people to live in fear ever since the pandemic began in 2020.

---

[81] "Coronavirus Death Toll May Reach 100,000 to 240,000 in U.S. Despite Actions, Officials Say," New York Times, March 31, 2020, https://www.nytimes.com/2020/03/31/us/politics/ coronavirus-death-toll-united-states.html.

[82] C.H. Spurgeon, Prayer (Whitaker House, 2001), 125.

Chapter 21

Hope: The Anchor of the Soul

The only way to manage stress from any disease, including COVID-19 and others, is to activate hope. During any sickness (but especially a pandemic), we cannot afford to live while lugging around a load of stress. Diseases, pain, and disabilities are real. So is the fear of death. All of these inflict tormenting thoughts on our minds that negatively affect our body, soul, and spirit. I approach all my patients as real people with this three-part make-up. I try to be fair in all approaches to people with the truth in my heart and mind, just as my Creator cares for me. He is the One who brings healing and comfort, and restores joy in my life. That increases my faith and hope, which further reduces stress.

Isaiah reassured us that God sent Jesus Christ, His Son when the prophet wrote these notable words: "To console those who mourn in Zion, to give them beauty for ashes, the oil of joy for mourning, the garment of praise for the spirit of heaviness; that they may be called trees of righteousness, the planting of the LORD, that He may be glorified" (Isa. 61:3). Jesus is the answer to all problems in the world and the only hope that we can have for our physical and spiritual health. Belief in Him makes an eternal impact.

I like research, scientific evidence, and the results from such studies. Still, I must acknowledge the limitations I saw in our capability to control the pandemic—with consequences for the entire world. Even with the highest expertise and the most advanced technology, millions of people died unnecessarily during the pandemic. Even though they make a huge difference in people's lives, we do not have a 100 percent guarantee when it comes to combating any disease, despite all our varied skills, knowledge, and expertise.

After thirty years in the long-term care business, I can confidently state that more research is needed in every area of human suffering. I have treated patients with fifteen to twenty different medications on their medication lists, but who still continued to suffer from their chronic diseases and disabilities. Many finally died from those diseases and nobody knows exactly how much pain they endured. We only assume that they had less pain and less discomfort with the intervention of medical experts. The only lasting hope someone can have is in Jesus Christ, the Messiah who saves our being and anchors our soul to God's power and presence. As the writer of Hebrews says: "This hope we have as an anchor of the soul, both sure and steadfast, and which enters the Presence behind the veil, where the forerunner has entered for us, even Jesus, having become High Priest forever according to the order of Melchizedek" (Heb. 6:19–20).

When we believe in our heart that:

- Jesus Christ is the Son of God
- That He died on the cross for our sins and shed His blood to save the world
- That God raised Him from the dead, and
- We confess with our mouth that He is Lord over our life, opening our heart and letting Him take residence in us through the power of the Holy Spirit by faith ...

He becomes our eternal hope, as stated in Colossians: "To them God willed to make known what are the riches of the glory of this mystery among the Gentiles: which is Christ in you, the hope of glory" (Col. 1:27).

Supernatural Wisdom

Without hope in God's supernatural power, efforts using only physical and intellectual resources to prevent the spread of viruses and prescribe treatments are limited. We must recognize that we cannot trust in human wisdom, knowledge, and understanding during a pandemic time. We have proved that we are incompetent to prevent disaster in the world in the face of the Covid virus—the cruel enemy of our body, soul, and spirit. This virus damaged our entire world physically, emotionally, socially, economically, and ethically. Such overwhelming destruction should cause us to turn to a Higher Power for help; as Proverbs advises: "Trust in the LORD with all your heart, and lean not on your own understanding; in all your ways acknowledge Him, and He shall direct your paths" (Prov. 3:5–6).

Hope increases when we acknowledge God's supernatural wisdom in every discovery we make through research. We will know true joy and peace when we recognize that every gift is from Him through the Holy Spirit. This Spirit is real and at work on this planet according to the apostle James: "Every good gift and every perfect gift is from above, and comes down from the Father of lights, with whom there is no variation or shadow of turning" (James 1:17). We did not bring anything into this world. Our capability to design studies, for understanding and interpreting scientific results, and our ability to memorize and remember information is from God. He is Jehovah Elohim, the Creator of the heavens and earth.

Through the power of the Holy Spirit, we receive wisdom, inspiration, and discernment. We become knowledgeable in our world to function as we do through our actions. Everything we know—I mean everything on this planet since its creation—is from God the Father through His precious Son, Jesus. As Paul wrote in his letter to the church at Ephesus, it was his prayer "that the God of our Lord Jesus Christ, the Father of glory, may give to you the spirit of wisdom and revelation in the knowledge of Him, the eyes of your understanding being enlightened; that you may know what is the hope of His calling, what are the riches of the glory of His inheritance in the saints, and what is the exceeding greatness of His power toward us who believe, according to the working of His mighty power" (Eph. 1:17–19).

Promises for Healing

The key to healing is to listen for God's voice and obey by doing what is right in His sight. In Exodus 15:26 God promised, "If you diligently heed the voice of the LORD your God and do what is right in His sight, give ear to His commandments and keep all His statutes, I will put none of the diseases on you which I have brought on the Egyptians. For I am the LORD who heals you." Trust the Word of God and have faith in Christ. He is moved with compassion and wants to heal every suffering person when we come to Him with childlike faith.

The Bible tells us that Jesus was a remarkable, revolutionary-style leader. Instead of laying heavy burdens on people like the Pharisees who took Ten Commandments and turned them into a staggering list of 613 legalistic, onerous rules, He came to set people free, heal them, and grant them a new life. The Gospel of Matthew describes how: "Jesus went through all the towns and villages, teaching in their synagogues, proclaiming the good news of the kingdom and healing every disease and sickness. When he saw the crowds, he had compassion on them, because they were harassed and helpless, like sheep without a shepherd" (Matt. 9:35–36 NIV).

The Lord died on the cross for our sins, so that our souls can be saved through His suffering and wounds, and so we can receive healing. In words he didn't fully understand at the time he wrote them, the prophet Isaiah said, "But he was pierced for our transgressions, he was crushed for our iniquities; the punishment that brought us peace was on him, and by his wounds we are healed" (Isa. 53:5 NIV). When we seek God's forgiveness for our sins, He is faithful to forgive all our sins and to heal our diseases. This is why King David wrote in the Psalms: "Praise the LORD, my soul; all my inmost being, praise his holy name. Praise the LORD, my soul, and forget not all his benefits—who forgives all your sins and heals all your diseases" (Ps. 103:1–3 NIV). Forgiveness of our sins is the key to healing for all our diseases past, present, and future.

Divine Protection

As a health care professional for three decades, and a general practitioner providing direct care to thousands of patients with acute and chronic illnesses—and seeing so many dying over the years—I know that we have only one hope. That hope is found in God and His Son's blood to cover us and to protect us in the shadow of His wings. I love the first two verses of Psalm 91, which say, "He who dwells in the secret place of the Most High shall abide under the shadow of the Almighty. I will say of the LORD, 'He is my refuge and my fortress; my God, in Him I will trust." I often used those words to encourage myself when I endured struggles and fear during the pandemic.

I echo Stephen Strang's words from his book on how the pandemic was affecting Christians: "I believe strongly that God has given us a powerful and miraculous immune system to fight off the possible trillions of viruses in the world. Many of today's processed foods and GMOs directly target our immune system. This only solidifies the case to build our immunity and practice wisdom in our eating habits. Dr. Colbert told me that, first of all, as Christians we must approach this pandemic with faith and not fear. We must pray Psalm 91 over ourselves and our families: 'Surely He shall deliver you from the snare of the hunter and from the deadly pestilence' (Ps. 91:3 MEV). 'Read the Word out loud over yourself and your family every day, and then receive that word by faith and don't live in fear,' Colbert said. I would add that we should plead the blood of Jesus over ourselves and our loved ones each day and truly put on the full armor of God. After all, in many ways this is what we have trained for."[83]

From my experience as a Christian who lived in a communist country for more than three decades and a believer in God's Word, I encourage patients to pray the following verses boldly:

- "Keep me as the apple of Your eye; hide me under the shadow of Your wings" (Ps. 17:8).

[83] God, Trump, and COVID-19, 62.

- "The LORD is my rock and my fortress and my deliverer; my God, my strength, in whom I will trust; my shield and the horn of my salvation, my stronghold" (Ps. 18:4).
- "The name of the LORD is a strong tower; the righteous run to it and are safe" (Prov. 18:10).
- "My soul, wait silently for God alone, For my expectation is from Him. He only is my rock and my salvation; He is my defense; I shall not be moved. In God is my salvation and my glory; the rock of my strength, and my refuge, is in God. Trust in Him at all times, you people; pour out your heart before Him; God is a refuge for us. Selah" (Ps. 62:5–8).

This is how I overcame fear during communism—by having a lifestyle of prayer and believing God's living Word and His promises for my life, and this is how I face fear from the enemy of my soul during current times.

When authorities forced us to practice social distancing, we got nearer to God in His spiritual realm through prayer. When forced to wear masks, we raised our voices to God through the Holy Spirit, drawing closer to our Creator. I am sharing with you, dear readers, so you know that our battle is not against people but spiritual evil: "For we do not wrestle against flesh and blood, but against principalities, against powers, against the rulers of the darkness of this age, against spiritual hosts of wickedness in the heavenly places" (Eph. 6:12). Fear is the enemy of our body, soul, and spirit, seeking to create a second pandemic in the world. Only through faith can we overcome fear and its consequences. Because all things shall pass away, we must be people waiting for the Lord to return in faith.

Church is Essential

It is essential to belong to a church to be part of the body of Christ. We need to be part of a local church as we join with the worldwide church known as the body of Christ, to improve our immune system physically and spiritually. In doing so, we receive spiritual food and encouragement in the same way every cell in the physical body receives nourishment. Church is a place where people worship God, the Creator of the universe, together in the Spirit—a place where people of faith assemble for fellowship and gain a sense of belonging. It is where their spiritual needs are satisfied and the joy of the Lord is restored in their soul.

For their physical and spiritual health, people need to communicate with each other face to face, as they interact, socialize, and find support. A church is a "spiritual clinic" where people's souls get restored and emotions healed when they are experiencing psychological distress. I am writing in the hope that we the people will learn from our past mistakes and not close churches down again. During a pandemic, the worst possible action to take is closing houses of worship so humans are depleted of God's mighty Presence at the very time when they need Him the most. Other measures can be implemented during a pandemic. Groups of people can take turns watching facilities throughout the week, but the church should stay open in the same way the ER is open twenty-four hours a day, seven days a week.

God created humans to worship Him. We see throughout the Bible that worship is essential for God to be present in the midst of a congregation. "Then the LORD said to Moses, 'Go to Pharaoh and say to him, "This is what the LORD, the God of the Hebrews, says: 'Let my people go, so that they may worship me'"' (Ex. 9:1 NIV). God knew that we were created for worship so He could present Himself in our midst. As we must have food daily to sustain the body, so we must have spiritual food available twenty-four hours a day. With no spiritual food, the soul will die. During the pandemic many of us sensed persecution at every level, physically and spiritually. This caused emotional suffering and spiritual damages to our spirits, souls, and bodies.

Ironically, when numerous state and/or local governments placed heavy restrictions on worship gatherings or closed down churches, they allowed liquor stores to remain open as "essential businesses." Yet in early 2025, outgoing US Surgeon General Dr. Vivek Murthy released a new advisory on alcohol consumption and increased cancer risk. In a statement, he said that alcohol represents the third leading preventable cause of cancer, after tobacco and obesity.

"Alcohol is a well-established, preventable cause of cancer responsible for about 100,000 cases of cancer and 20,000 cancer deaths annually in the United States—greater than the 13,500 alcohol-associated traffic crash fatalities per year in the US—yet the majority of Americans are unaware of this risk," Murthy said. "This Advisory lays out steps we can all take to increase awareness of alcohol's cancer risk and minimize harm."[84]

Maybe during the next pandemic, we should close liquor stores while encouraging people to go to church.

---

84 "U.S. Surgeon General Issues New Advisory on Link Between Alcohol and Cancer Risk," US Department of Health and Human Services, January 3, 2025, https://www.hhs.gov/about/news/2025/01/03/us-surgeon-general-issues-new-advisory-link-alcohol-cancer-risk.html.

Chapter 22

Encouragement for Those Who Mourn

"He heals the brokenhearted and binds up their wounds" (Ps. 147:3).

"For I consider that the sufferings of this present time are not worthy to be compared with the glory which shall be revealed in us" (Rom. 8:18).

Scriptures like the two above can serve as salve on the wounds of those who are still hurting after the loss of loved ones to the COVID-19 virus. During the pandemic, I heard news as never before of younger people dying in every corner of this planet. The emotional pain of separation through death is real and sometimes unbearable. Coronavirus restrictions accentuated that pain. Family members were often not allowed to participate in the burial ceremony of their loved ones, which added to their emotional pain and created higher stress levels. In turn, that increased their risk for more physical diseases.

To be able to bear that emotional pain and avoid depression from prolonged feelings of sadness, one must run to God's Word. Only by filling our hearts with the Holy Spirit's power can we find comfort through God's promises. As Romans says, "May the God of hope fill you with all joy and peace in believing, so that by the power of the Holy Spirit you may abound in hope" (Rom. 15:13 ESV). God in heaven is the one and only Being who can heal the brokenhearted and bind those deep wounds created by the painful separation of death.

We must always hope in God's promises. We must believe that He is breathing the breath of life into us, even in the most difficult and impossible of circumstances. And that He will make us live in the same way He breathed on "dry bones" and made them live, as described in Ezekiel 37. While this is a long passage, it is a powerful illustration of the supernatural power of the Spirit of God who makes impossible situations possible:

"The hand of the LORD came upon me and brought me out in the Spirit of the LORD, and set me down in the midst of the valley; and it was full of bones. Then He caused me to pass by them all around, and behold, there were very many in the open valley; and indeed they were very dry. And He said to me, 'Son of man, can these bones live?'

"So I answered, 'O Lord GOD, You know.'

"Again He said to me, 'Prophesy to these bones, and say to them, "O dry bones, hear the word of the Lord! Thus says the Lord GOD to these bones: 'Surely I will cause breath to enter into you, and you shall live. I will put sinews on you and bring flesh upon you, cover you with skin and put breath in you; and you shall live. Then you shall know that I am the LORD.'

"So I prophesied as I was commanded; and as I prophesied, there was a noise, and suddenly a rattling; and the bones came together, bone to bone. Indeed, as I looked, the sinews and the flesh came upon them, and the skin covered them over; but there was no breath in them.

"Also He said to me, 'Prophesy to the breath, prophesy, son of man, and say to the breath, Thus says the Lord GOD: Come from the four winds, O breath, and breathe on these slain, that they may live.' So I prophesied as He commanded me, and breath came into them, and they lived, and stood upon their feet, an exceedingly great army.

"Then He said to me, 'Son of man, these bones are the whole house of Israel. They indeed say, 'Our bones are dry, our hope is lost, and we ourselves are cut off!' Therefore prophesy and say to them, 'Thus says the Lord GOD: "Behold, O My people, I will open your graves and cause you to come up from your graves, and bring you into the land of Israel. Then you shall know that I am the LORD, when I have opened your graves, O My people, and brought you up from your graves. I will put My Spirit in you, and you shall live, and I will place you in your own land. Then you shall know that I, the LORD, have spoken it and performed it," says the LORD'" (Ezek. 37:1–14).

Reviving Dead Bones

As in ancient times, during the pandemic all nations on earth became a death valley full of "dead bones" because an invisible enemy stole their joy. Fear of COVID-19 affected the entire world and crushed the spirit of humanity. This caused anxiety and depression, which brought more physical and spiritual disease and premature death. Without joy, the bones of humanity became dry and crippled people's lives. We pray that the catastrophes from COVID-19, including banning early treatment in primary care settings, will never happen again to humanity. NEVER AGAIN.

As I mentioned in chapter 8, Proverbs says, "A cheerful heart is good medicine, but a crushed spirit dries up the bones" (Prov. 17:22 NIV). God wants us to have cheerful hearts. He wants to breathe His breath of life and supernatural love into all of us in order for us to be able to live, physically and spiritually. In this way, we can assist, serve, and comfort others with the comfort we have received. God's desire is that we know His Holy Spirit is real. He wants us to know that He can breathe His Spirit on us, His people, and we can live in this land to again see the goodness of God in the land of the living—to recognize that *He* is the great *I AM*. He is Jehovah Shammah, the God who is present in every moment of our lives to meet all our needs.

Only a holy God can restore the joy of our soul that can bring healing and restoration. Without the joy of salvation, nations will continue to dry up and become like a valley of dried bones. Our hearts must be filled with hope, joy, and peace when fear of COVID-19 or other viruses that arise in the future threaten to paralyze us. Our spiritual life is affected by fear and increased stress from worries and worldly concerns, which affects our spiritual health. During the coronavirus pandemic, I heard many times: "I have difficulty breathing." Through the power of the Holy Spirit and the promises of His Word we can breathe again.

The Bible gives us clear instructions and guidance on how to behave in our era with the most advanced technology, best experts, and advanced science. And how to do so with excellence in our daily lives: "Finally, brothers, whatever is true, whatever is honorable, whatever is just, whatever is pure, whatever is lovely, whatever is commendable, if there is any excellence, if there is anything worthy of praise, think about these things" (Phil. 4:8 ESV).

God, the Creator of the universe, gave us all things that pertain to life and excellence to help us escape the world's corruption. As the apostle Peter wrote: "His divine power has granted to us all things that pertain to life and godliness, through the knowledge of him who called us to his own glory and excellence, by which he has granted to us his precious and very great promises, so that through them you may become partakers of the divine nature, having escaped from the corruption that is in the world because of sinful desire" (2 Peter 1:3-4 ESV).

Creator of Life

Scripture describes the wonderfully unique and awesome ways in which God the Creator fashioned us for this world. Namely, to follow His purpose for our lives here on earth: "So God created man in His own image; in the image of God He created him; male and female He created them" (Gen. 1:27). In Psalm 139, David wrote: "For You formed my inward parts; You covered me in my mother's womb. I will praise You, for I am fearfully and wonderfully made; marvelous are Your works, and that my soul knows very well" (Ps. 139:13–14). As I wrote in my book, *Created in His Image with Unique Purpose*, "The human body is built with the most sophisticated, detailed built-in features and extremely complex connections of body, soul, and spirit with thoughts, emotions, and feelings! ... The purpose of God for the creation of humankind is greater than our mind can perceive, understand, and comprehend. Everyone has a destiny, with gifts and potential inside, with a purpose."[85] I realized that because of God's unique purpose in creation, each person is different—even in developing symptoms from diseases caused by viruses—and had a different clinical presentation after contracting the COVID-19 virus because of our uniqueness as God's creation.

So every single person developed different symptoms from the invisible enemy as they fought this unpredictable virus. They needed to be treated as soon as possible and prescribed prophylactic treatments, which many doctors proved work to prevent people from dying from COVID-19. (See all studies and protocols mentioned earlier; more are yet to be developed).

Sin in the world is another "invisible enemy" that produces spiritual diseases. As a strong believer in the power of the living Word of God, I have learned over the years that people are healed physically and spiritually (as Dr. Crandall put it) through the best of Christ and the best of medicine. Many Christian doctors and general practitioners have proven this true in their practices. Sometimes doctors and specialists have no control over a disease; it is beyond their knowledge and expertise.

When people are not healed in the body but have a restored soul and spiritual health, they then move to their eternal home. It is a place prepared by the Lord for those who believe in Him. They will glorify the Lord, with the cloud of witnesses who are waiting for all who remain on earth to join them one day to give glory to our Father forever and ever and ever. We are assured by His living Word: "Most assuredly, I say to you, he who hears My word and believes in Him who sent Me has everlasting life, and shall not come into judgment, but has passed from death into life" (John 5:24).

As we wait for this eternal passage, God is also waiting patiently for people and nations to return and come to Him in

---

[85] Dr. Rodica Malos, Created in His Image with Unique Purpose: Science and Beyond (Trilogy Publishing, 2021), 27 and 44.

repentance. Because He is the essence of love and mercy, He does not want anyone to perish. Peter describes this in his letter: "The Lord is not slow in keeping his promise, as some understand slowness. Instead he is patient with you, not wanting anyone to perish, but everyone to come to repentance" (2 Peter 3:9 NIV).

God is holy and is asking His creation to be holy. Living in an attitude of humility and righteousness is God's heart desire for every nation. As Proverbs says, "Righteousness exalts a nation, but sin is a reproach to any people" (Prov. 14:34). God calls us to repentance and prayer for the nation and the city where we live in order to enjoy peaceful lives. As the prophet Jeremiah wrote: "Also, seek the peace and prosperity of the city to which I have carried you into exile. Pray to the LORD for it, because if it prospers, you too will prosper" (Jer. 29:7 NIV).

Self-Evaluation

Today is a great opportunity to reassess your relationship with Jesus, the Lamb of God. The Christ who died on the cross for the sins of the entire world and rose again on the third day is just waiting for each sinner to confess their sins and to receive Him as their personal Savior.

Without Jesus Christ there is no salvation, no meaning to life on earth, and no eternal life in heaven. Jesus is the only way to heaven, which He pointed out to Thomas as the disciples gathered around Him once for an extended discussion: "Thomas said to Him, 'Lord, we do not know where You are going, and how can we know the way?' Jesus said to him, 'I am the way, the truth, and the life. No one comes to the Father except through Me'" (John 14:5–6).

Jesus Christ is the only hope for our sins to be forgiven. The only hope of enjoying eternal life with Him in heaven, after this life on earth passes away. Each one of us needs Jesus to wash our sins away, because we are all sinners. As Paul wrote to the church at Rome: "For all have sinned and fall short of the glory of God, being justified freely by His grace through the redemption that is in Christ Jesus, whom God set forth as a propitiation by His blood, through faith, to demonstrate His righteousness, because in His forbearance God had passed over the sins that were previously committed, to demonstrate at the present time His righteousness, that He might be just and the justifier of the one who has faith in Jesus" (Rom. 3:23–26).

I am writing this example of a prayer you can say to receive Jesus Christ into your heart. When you do, you can receive forgiveness of your sins and start a new life on earth that will lead to eternal life in heaven. This means you will be with the Lord forever and ever after this temporary life ends:

"Father God in heaven, I have sinned against You. I recognize and confess all my sins, from when I was born until today. Cleanse me with the precious holy blood that was shed by the Lamb of God, Your Son, Jesus Christ. Now Lord Jesus, come into my heart through the power of the Holy Spirit and be my personal Lord and Savior. Transform my life. Today I want to start a new life with You, Jesus, who died on the cross for my sins, and was resurrected on the third day and ascended to heaven. You are sitting at the right hand of the Father, the Creator of the universe, to intercede for me, my family, and the entire world. Thank You for forgiving my sins and for saving me. Thank You for giving me eternal life so I can be with You forever and ever. From now on I want to live for you. In Jesus's name I pray, amen."

Changing the Atmosphere

The atmosphere in your brain changes when you pray. The words you speak in prayer have the power to change your mind and transform your life. That powerful prayer will change your "spiritual DNA," instantly changing your thoughts and releasing a healthy amount of neurotransmitters. To quote from my book, *Find Your Peace*, "When you and pray and enter into the presence of God, great joy will flood your soul. You have had an audience with the CEO of the universe! When you pray, the presence of God brings you peace, even in the middle of a 'storm.' God uses storms to wake us up, to seek His presence." [86]

We know that each one of us on earth will die one day and must face God's judgment. Hebrews spells that out: "Just as people are destined to die once, and after that to face judgment, so Christ was sacrificed once to take away the sins of many; and he will appear a second time, not to bear sin, but to bring salvation to those who are waiting for him" (Heb. 9:27–28 NIV). And in his letter to the Corinthians, the apostle Paul noted, "For he says, 'In the time of my favor I heard you, and in the day of salvation I helped you.' I tell you, now is the time of God's favor, now is the day of salvation" (2 Cor. 6:2 NIV). The day of leaving this planet is the most important day in each person's life. It is important to be ready for that day, because none of us knows when our time will be over. That is what happened to millions on the earth during the pandemic. Today is the day to receive God's salvation.

[86] Find Your Peace, 237.

Conclusion

Never Again

Persecution for telling the truth is real. The Lord gave us a warning about persecution almost two thousand years ago through Paul's statement that "all who desire to live godly in Christ Jesus will suffer persecution" (2 Tim. 3:12). Throughout my life, I learned from persecution—from the communists back in Romania and in the US during the pandemic—that the highest honor and call for every human being is to stand up for the truth and to fight for freedom, regardless of persecution. The truth guarantees our freedom: "And you shall know the truth, and the truth shall make you free" (John 8:32).

During Romania's communist regime, the government marginalized, threatened, intimidated, and restricted Christians like myself from using their rights to live a normal life. Secret police kept believers under constant surveillance. We were not allowed to visit family and friends outside the country, simply because of our values, beliefs, high moral standards, and speaking the truth. Christians were not allowed to own or openly read the Bible or Christian literature. We weren't allowed to talk to anyone about our values, visions, hopes, faith in God and His Word, or our dreams. Those courageous enough to "buck the system" were investigated for long hours. Some lost their jobs or were imprisoned for years while their families lived under threats, intimidation, humiliation, and persecution from the authorities.

Persecution for the truth was real then. It is real today. Fighting for freedom is everyone's duty to prevent communism from resurfacing, along with dictatorship, totalitarianism, globalism, and the consequences for generations of losing our freedom. If that happens, our children and their children and their children's children will have to suffer, just as we suffered in Romania. The truth is that during the pandemic, dictatorship obstructed free thinking in medicine. In primary care settings we were not allowed to treat suffering people; if we dared to do so, we were threatened with loss of our license, professional standing, and career.

The license revocation decision by the Oregon nursing board shocked me. As I mentioned in chapter 1, this action devastated me, indicating that my critical thinking and judgment skills were of no value. My three decades of practice were lost, along with freedom in medicine. The state declared that using my license to benefit the most vulnerable patients—the underprivileged, the poor, and ethnic and racial minorities—wasn't important. Nor was my work with a community clinic with the mission to provide care with the love of Jesus Christ. And, to be the feet and hands of Jesus in our community, using the best scientific evidence available at that time.

Reflecting on that nightmare my heart cried out, "Never again will we allow that to happen to suffering patients." I felt like I were fighting the Goliath of our time, but I also knew that David won the battle with the giant because he had God on his side. With that picture in mind I began the battle in medicine. The overwhelming news of COVID-19 spread via the local, national, and international news. It aired on TV, over radio and the internet, through social media, newspapers, at the grocery store, and countless offices. Everyone was literally talking about it and as they did, fear escalated.

Pinned by Sadness

No matter who I talked to—family members, neighbors, friends, pastors, doctors, legislators, lay persons, or professional people—both here and abroad, I sensed the sadness pinning everyone's thoughts to one term: COVID-19. It would dictate our everyday existence for the rest of our lives. Because of my background in medicine, I knew the consequences of fear and sadness: stirring up negative thoughts, causing a shift in neurotransmitters and decreasing serotonin, dopamine, endorphins, melatonin, and other neurochemicals. That leads to depression and all its consequences. The battle is real in our mind, waged by thoughts of fear and despair.

As I mentioned in chapter 7, thoughts of fear can take up "real estate" in our brain, with billions of neurons and repeating thoughts of fear surging through our mind. They will control it, causing the immune system to weaken and not be able to fight COVID-19 or other viruses, both those present and others yet to come. When our immunity is down, a virus can cause more damage to our body, soul, and spirit. I knew that the only way to overcome fear is by faith, which is the uncontestable antidote for every fearful situation, and that faith comes by hearing. As Dr. Simone Gold (who I mentioned a couple times previously) says: "Fear is like radioactivity: once released, it filters into everything. But we can stop being afraid by choosing to live joyfully in hope." [87]

I knew from experience that only the living Word of God can help banish fear, reassuring us that He is with us in the most difficult times: "And the LORD, He is the One who goes before you. He will be with you, He will not leave you nor forsake you; do not fear nor be dismayed" (Deut. 31:8). When we embrace this truth, sadness is replaced by joy. Joy is one of the most powerful emotions for bringing healing to our body, spirit, and soul. It is the antidote for sadness and depression. The reward mechanism in our brain is activated when we are full of joy and dopamine is released, improving our motivation for the activities of daily living and everyday life.

To dissipate thoughts of fear and sadness during the pandemic proved extremely difficult, especially when patients and their families were facing such an aggressive enemy. Throughout the pandemic, people had endless questions because of the uncertainties they faced. We directed them to the resources available and to professional health care providers, doctors, and nurses working in the health fields that

---

[87] *I Do Not Consent*, 72.

were knowledgeable. These experts informed people of how to get relief from fear, anxiety, and depression. When I found the solution with early interventions from brave Frontline Doctors, it aroused hope in my soul and spirit, shifting the atmosphere in my mind. Hope alleviated fear. I started to share this solution immediately with discouraged patients to bring hope and joy into their lives.

Biblical Promises

After all, this was a time when we could not afford to live with overwhelming stress. Disease, pain, and disabilities are real, as is death. The fear arising from these factors torment our minds. Thank God that we have Him to relieve us of fear. He is the One who brings healing and comfort, restores joy, and increases faith and hope, which reduces stress. Isaiah reassures us that God sent Jesus Christ, His Son, "to console those who mourn in Zion, to give them beauty for ashes, the oil of joy for mourning, the garment of praise for the spirit of heaviness; that they may be called trees of righteousness, the planting of the LORD, that He may be glorified" (Isa. 61:3).

Isaiah echoes other scriptures that brim with promises, like:

- Exodus 15:26: "If you diligently heed the voice of the LORD your God and do what is right in His sight, give ear to His commandments and keep all His statutes, I will put none of the diseases on you which I have brought on the Egyptians. For I am the LORD who heals you."
- Exodus 23:25: " So you shall serve the LORD your God, and He will bless your bread and your water. And I will take sickness away from the midst of you."
- Deuteronomy 7:15: "And the LORD will take away from you all sickness, and will afflict you with none of the terrible diseases of Egypt which you have known, but will lay them on all those who hate you."

- Proverbs 19:8: "He who gets wisdom loves his own soul; he who keeps understanding will find good."

Given such promises and the reality of the spiritual battle involved with the pandemic, the Holy Spirit prompted me to share my experiences and those of my patients so that we may get insights in the event of another pandemic. Or, for other difficult situations that may arise. Sometimes, we all learn from mistakes, especially when we go through uncertain circumstances. We cannot be ignorant of our past experiences and the knowledge and resources available at a crucial moment to help us move on. During hard times, we can have the peace that passes all understanding when we draw wisdom from above.

In chapter 2, I detailed the array of doctors around the world who helped save thousands upon thousands of lives through early treatments. It likely saved an even greater number by preventing the fear that could have created a second pandemic. While this great news brought much hope to the world, leaders and those in authority in the health care system refused to learn of ways to save lives. Using dictatorial methods, they persecuted those who sacrificed their profession and their lives to save others. They restricted doctors from using their knowledge, expertise, and scientific evidence, and instructed pharmacists to reject prescriptions for off-label purposes, even though the FDA has recognized this as safe.

In his book about the COVID-19 cover-up, Robert F. Kennedy Jr. noted that "during the COVID crisis, (some manipulated) the science to suppress safe and miraculously effective early treatment remedies. The fraudulent Solidarity study provided extremely high, even lethal doses of hydroxychloroquine to elderly patients to 'prove' its dangerousness."[88]

He also mentioned the defamation of the safe medications by "researchers" using fraudulent databases for propaganda, spreading disinformation and hindering safe medications that could have saved

---

[88] *The Wuhan Cover-Up and the Terrifying Bioweapons Arms Race*, 633.

countless lives if used early in the disease process. Kennedy also stated that on May 22, 2020, well-known British medical journal The Lancet published a fabricated study discrediting hydroxychloroquine and chloroquine. The bottom line, he wrote, was that the Covid patients given the drugs were supposedly dying at higher rates and suffering more heart-related problems than others stricken with the virus who went untreated.

"The World Health Organization cited the study as a justification for ending its clinical trials of HCQ," Kennedy said. "Three European nations outlawed its use for COVID-19. Angry questions about gross inconsistencies in The Lancet study by hundreds of doctors and scientists worldwide forced an investigation that revealed that the researchers had based their consequential defamations of hydroxychloroquine on a giant database that didn't actually exist. The dataset underlying that study turned out to be the invention of a small Illinois-based 'medical education' company. The Surgisphere Corporation had a curiously comprised handful of staff, including a science fiction writer and an adult content model.

"Horton admitted that the paper, since retracted, was a 'fabrication' and 'a monumental fraud'; Surgisphere's CEO went into hiding, and the company disappeared from the Internet. The New England Journal of Medicine, which has a similar quiver of conflicts, had to simultaneously retract its own article, also published in May, based on the same fraudulent database. Dr. Horton and NEJM's editor in chief, Dr. Eric Rubin, admitted to The New York Times that the studies should never have appeared in their publications. America's Frontline Doctors commented that '[t]he sheer number and magnitude of the things that went wrong or missing are too enormous to attribute to mere incompetence.' They also opined, 'What's incredible is that the editors of these esteemed journals still have a job.'"[89]

Earlier, I mentioned comments from Dr. Robert Malone's book, Lies My Gov't Told Me. In another section, he wrote: "We could

---

[89] Ibid., 264.

have put an end to this pandemic and saved countless lives if many more physicians had spoken up in their individual institutions, prioritizing early treatment approaches guided by the precautionary principle and sound risk-benefit decision making. Instead, physician leaders in countless institutions allowed public health agencies and institutions to implement a rigid, top-down approach to treatment, threatening physicians with loss of their livelihoods if they didn't follow their preordained protocols. The physicians' cowardice in staying silent, while patients suffered and died."[90]

In addition to the millions of patients who died, other doctors and nurses who dared to stand up for the truth and sacrifice their lives also died on the frontlines of the pandemic. At the International Crisis Summit I attended in Bucharest in November of 2023, they pictured the first UK doctors to die of COVID-19; more than a dozen photographs appeared onscreen.

The refusal of medical authorities to permit early treatment to save lives at any cost still grips my heart. During the pandemic, the inhuman behavior of dictators banning treatment for patients suffering from Covid and the persecution of doctors who saved lives shook humanity to the core. It also led me to write this book as a reminder to not let this kind of disaster to ever happen again. I repeat what I said in chapter 22: NEVER AGAIN.

When I think about the disaster of patients running desperately from clinic to clinic to find a doctor and from pharmacy to pharmacy to find the medications to treat the symptoms that threatened their very existence, I also think about my Jewish grandfather. About what he felt when he ran in desperation to find a hiding place to save his life and the lives of his children during the Holocaust—and what he would tell his children and grandchildren about that atrocity. My father was only a child of twelve when he had to walk by himself from the city of Iasi in eastern Romania northwest to Dorohoi (a distance of more than ninety miles) to escape from those who were looking to arrest Jews

[90] *Lies My Gov't Told Me*, 102.

during this tragic time. What was going on in the mind of this young child desperately seeking a hiding place to escape the evil doers and death?

I came to the conclusion that faith triumphs over evil, even during the darkest moments in our lives. Evil happened right under our own eyes during the pandemic. Letting the virus take people's lives by denying them early treatment and thus destroying families, education, the economy, and mental health for generations was a reality, not a drill. I think of how Corrie ten Boom explained "the drill" in her book, The Hiding Place. How her father and his family practiced seeing how quickly they could hide Jewish citizens of Holland from the police and Gestapo who were arresting Jewish people and sending them to prison. There, most of them would die. She wrote that "this is what the past is for! Every experience God gives us, every person He puts in our lives is the perfect preparation for a future that only He can see."[91]

Maybe the pandemic was a drill; people's minds were filled with fear. But for the patients who came to the Christian clinic where I was able to save lives found the "hiding place" for those suffering with symptoms from Covid. The early treatments they received saved their lives in the same way Holocaust survivors accessed the secret refuge at Corrie ten Boom's home. As we move deeper into the twenty-first century, who knows what will happen next? Socialism and communism with would-be dictators, tyranny, and totalitarianism are knocking at the door. We need to wake up and be bold, and stand in the gap for our children and their children and future generations. The time is now. Every patient's life matters.

---

[91] Corrie ten Boom with Elizabeth and John Sherrill, *The Hiding Place*: 35th Anniversary Edition (Chosen Books, 2006), 12.

Physical and Spiritual Preparation

During the pandemic the virus found many people unprepared. People were completely misinformed about the disease's process and early interventions that saved lives. They did not know how to fight with an invisible enemy.

I had patients calling me late at night and even on weekends, desperate for help. One patient asked if I could let her borrow the medications I obtained from my doctor via telemedicine when I was sick. It saddened me that patients like her did not understand that I could not give someone medications from my own prescriptions. I said that I wanted to help, but if I shared my meds there wouldn't be enough for either of us. I advised her to contact the ER, but like so many patients she was sent home from the department with no treatment. So many were devastated that they had no treatment available and their symptoms were getting worse. I told her to go again and if she still couldn't get any treatment to try telemedicine to get treatment and supplies right away.

It still pains me to think of the terrible hardships patients endured because they were misinformed by authorities about early interventions. And, that doctors were unable to prescribe the right treatment because pharmacies were not allowed to fill off-label prescriptions, even if they did help patients with symptoms from COVID-19.

One night, a scripture came to mind about spiritual preparation for the return of Jesus Christ. The parable of the ten virgins (five foolish and five wise) waiting for the bridegroom appears in Matthew: "And at midnight a cry was heard: 'Behold, the bridegroom is coming; go out to meet him!' Then all those virgins arose and trimmed their lamps. And the foolish said to the wise, 'Give us some of your oil, for our lamps are going out.' But the wise answered, saying, 'No, lest there should not be enough for us and you; but go rather to those who sell, and buy for yourselves.' And while they went to buy, the bridegroom came, and those who were ready went in with him to the wedding; and the door was shut" (Matt. 25:6–10).

While here on planet earth, we need to be vigilant and prepared to have some reserves in our homes for emergencies. At our business we had to regularly conduct disaster preparedness training, since it was required for businesses in our area. You can take similar steps. Store up emergency food and water for disasters like the wildfires that struck the Los Angeles area in early 2025. Keep over-the-counter medications on hand and be wise with the use of any antibiotics or other medications. Do not use medications (especially antibiotics) without getting sound medical advice.

I think that everything that happens in the natural world also happens spiritually. So I emphasize the need for spiritual preparedness. When the rapture of the church, the bride, takes place we must be ready for this spiritual emergency. We must be prepared with our vessels filled with holy oil burning for the coming of our Lord and King. As for those who mourn the loved ones who have passed away, we must anchor our faith in the hope of God's promises and fully trust Him. As it is written in His living Word: "God will wipe away every tear from their eyes; there shall be no more death, nor sorrow, nor crying. There shall be no more pain, for the former things have passed away" (Rev. 21:4).

The bottom line is to always be ready. I repeat what General Mike Flynn says in the title of his 2024 documentary: "Deliver the truth, whatever the cost."[92] I just did. Now it is your turn.

[92] You can read more about it and purchase a copy at https://www.amazon.com/Flynn-Michael/dp/B0CT9JVB4F

About the Author

Born in Romania in a large family of nine children, Rodica Malos's family suffered under communist tyranny and oppression because of their Christian beliefs. Yet Rodica never lost her faith in the power of the Word of God, especially its ability to promote physical and spiritual health. Growing up in impoverished conditions and facing constant opposition, Rodica persevered and achieved a high level of education. After graduating from the Academy of Economic Science in Bucharest, she worked as an economist until leaving the country.

Arriving in the United States in 1990 with no English skills or finances, initially she earned a living as a caregiver for elderly nursing home patients. In 1992, she launched an at-home business offering foster care. Rodica also enrolled in medical studies and eventually earned several degrees, including a Doctor of Nursing Practice (DNP) from Oregon Health & Science University in Portland.

Her DNP is a PhD degree with clinical orientation and a focus on metabolic syndrome (hypertension, diabetes, dyslipidemia) in primary care practice. She also received clinical training, cardiology consulting, and training in internal medicine and general medicine primary care at various hospitals and medical facilities in the Portland area.

Rodica worked in the health care field for about three decades. She also practiced general medicine for more than twenty years, providing care to minorities, marginalized, the homeless, and other needy people, volunteering more than fifteen thousand hours at two community health clinics in Portland. With Agape Health Care, she provided care for minorities and others lacking access to the health care system. She also organized health fairs and free clinics in Portland and Romania.

She and her husband, Stelica, have been married for nearly four decades. They were the founders, co-CEOs, and operators of two Malos Adult Foster Homes and two memory care facilities. For approximately thirty years, Tabor Crest I and Tabor Crest II Memory Care provided physical, emotional, and spiritual care (including comfort care at the end of life) to thousands of elderly patients with multiple chronic conditions, including neurocognitive disorders and memory loss.

Dr. Malos is an international speaker and organizes and speaks at medical and Christian conferences in the US and other nations. As a board member at Star of Hope USA, she travels abroad and supports children with disabilities and their families financially, emotionally, and spiritually. She is the author of *Find Your Peace: Supernatural Solutions Beyond Science for Fear, Anxiety, and Depression* (2019); Created in His Image with Unique Purpose (2021); and COVID-19 & Post COVID-19: *Alleviate the Fear* (2021). Her website is http://rodicamalos.com.

Other Books by Dr. Rodica Malos

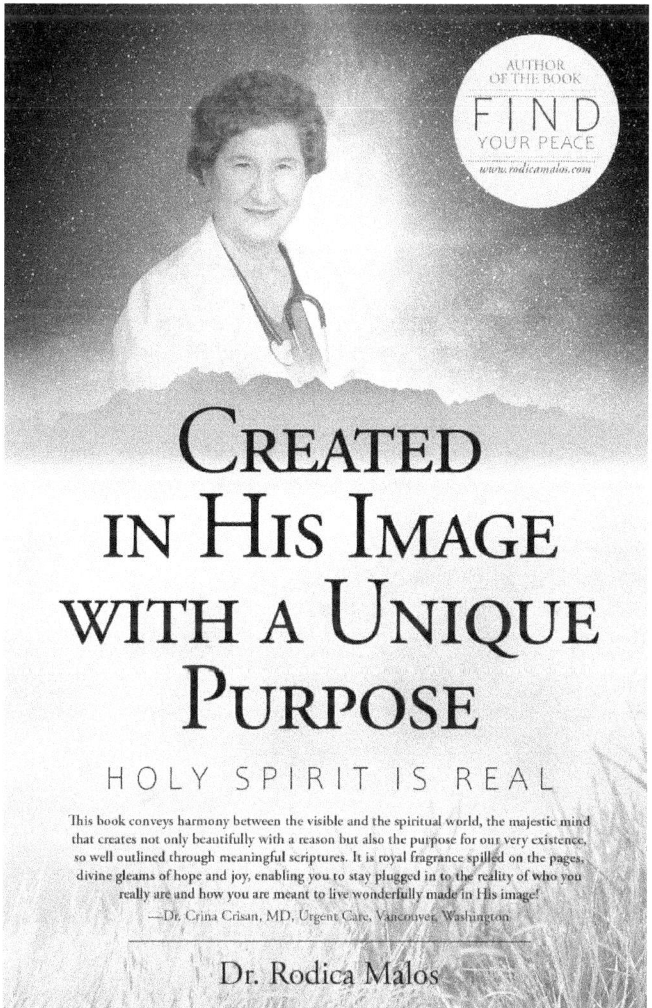

Other books written by Dr. Rodica Malos
available on Amazon.

FIND YOUR
PEACE

Supernatural Solutions Beyond Science for Fear, Anxiety, and Depression

RODICA MALOS, DNP

Other books written by Dr. Rodica Malos
available on Amazon.